Clean Eating Alice

THE
BODY
BIBLE

Thorsons
An imprint of HarperCollins*Publishers*
1 London Bridge Street
London SE1 9GF

www.harpercollins.co.uk

First published by Thorsons 2016

10 9 8 7 6 5 4

Photography © Philip Haynes: pages 4 (top, bottom right), 6, 23, 30, 135, 139,
141, 145–155, 159–170, 175–187, 191, 192, 194–205, 209, 210, 212–213;
© Martin Poole: pages 4 (bottom left), 36–41, 43, 47, 48, 53, 57, 58, 67, 68,
77, 78, 81, 85, 91, 93, 99, 103, 106, 114, 117, 118, 121, 122, 127, 129, 130, 133, 217.

Food styling: Kim Morphew
Prop styling: Wei Tang
Styling: Lucy Denver
Hair and make-up: Tahira Herold and Susanna Mota

A catalogue record of this book is available from the British Library

ISBN 978-0-00-816720-2

Printed and bound in Spain by Graficas Estella

MIX
Paper from
responsible sources
FSC www.fsc.org
FSC™ C007454

FSC™ is a non-profit international organisation established to promote the
responsible management of the world's forests. Products carrying the FSC
label are independently certified to assure consumers that they come from
forests that are managed to meet the social, economic and ecological needs
of present and future generations, and other controlled sources.

Find out more about HarperCollins and the environment at
www.harpercollins.co.uk/green

Clean Eating Alice

THE
BODY
BIBLE

Feel fit and fabulous
from the inside out

Thorsons

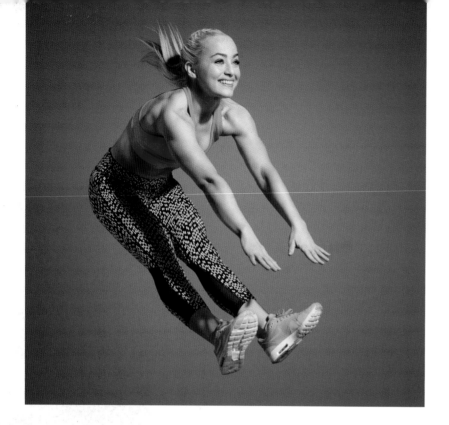
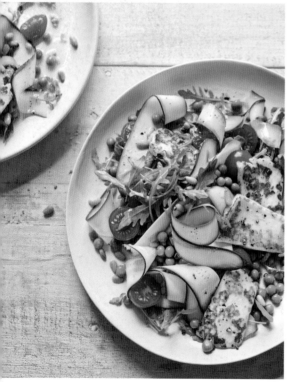
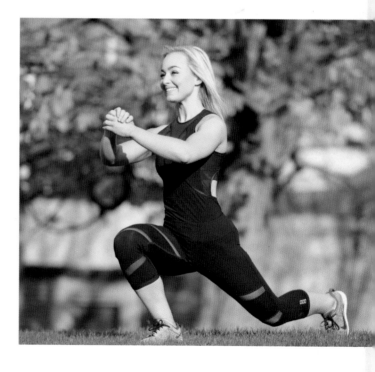

Contents

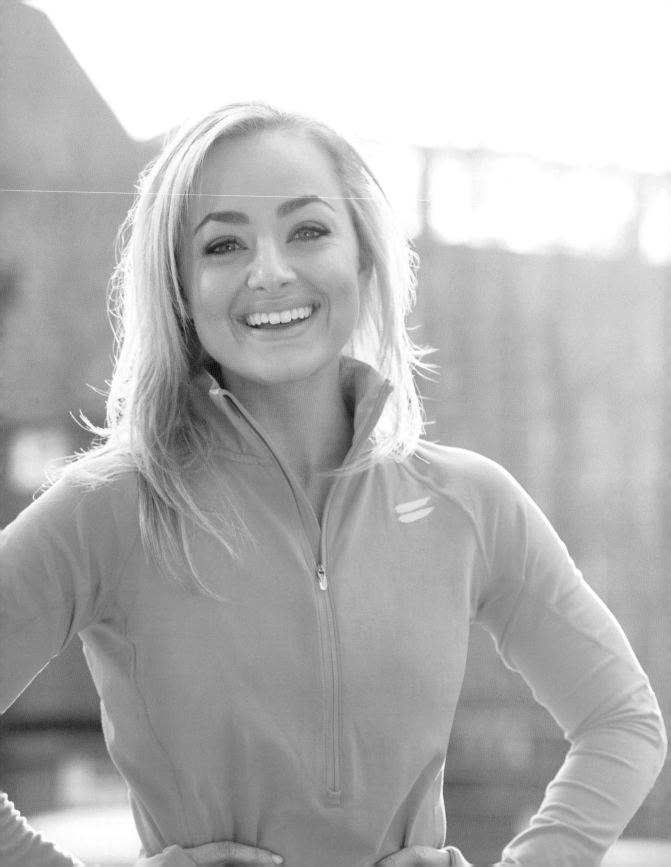

Dear Reader

Firstly, I'd like to say thank you for buying my book. Deciding to change your approach to eating and exercise takes huge courage and will require you to completely overhaul your previous concept of what a 'diet' should be. This book is about looking and feeling great inside and out. You will have to be disciplined and dedicated, but I promise: you will get out what you put in.

There are so many books out there at the moment that talk about 'clean eating'. The truth is that it is impossible to define one single meaning that is the same for everyone. For me it is simple: it is about eating nutrient-dense, whole foods to create, nourish and fuel a healthy mind and body.

When I began my journey I knew it wasn't a quick fix that I was after, that what I really needed was permanent change. In a world where everything is so instant and we have been conditioned to believe that a diet should have rapid results, we've lost the concept of understanding how to properly nourish our bodies to achieve long-term and sustainable change.

When I began my journey I knew it wasn't a quick fix that I was after, that what I really needed was permanent change.

Instead we see quick fixes like juice detoxes and stupidly low-calorie 'diets' as the fast-track way to what we perceive to be healthy. This had been the story of my life. I've done the 'no carbs after six o'clock' and the 'everything low fat, no fat' and, quite honestly, they made me feel completely the opposite of healthy. I simply felt, despite my best efforts, unhappy and unable to make any real difference to my physique.

I needed something so much more than that. I needed to be healthy and happy.

It's from this place that I decided that short-term measures just weren't going to cut it for me. I knew I needed something so much more than that. I needed to be healthy and happy.

So let's begin with HEALTHY.
Now, everyone's definition of healthy is different. As the saying goes: 'What's normal for the spider, is chaos for the fly.'

On day one, I got out my notepad (I'm such a list-maker) and wrote down everything that I wanted to achieve in terms of health. I'll be honest and say abs weren't even on my list! Nope, what I wanted was energy, muscular strength and definition, a good relationship with food where I didn't feel guilty for eating certain foods, a clear complexion and a greater understanding of how my body works.

What I wanted was energy, muscular strength and definition, a good relationship with food whereby I didn't feel guilty for eating certain foods, a clear complexion and a greater understanding of how my body works.

HAPPY
This wasn't something that I deliberately set out to discover, but as I started to enjoy food, love the gym and feel energized like never before, I realized that all aspects of my mindset were changing. I began to feel incredibly motivated in every area of my life. At college I found a new confidence in myself and started to really believe that I was good enough. At the gym I pushed myself to

gain strength. Overall, I felt calmer in the knowledge that I had taken control of a situation that had spiralled so out of control. It may sound obvious, but I cannot stress how clear it became that what I put into my body affected every single aspect of me, and overhauling my diet was absolutely pivotal in me changing not just physically, but mentally too.

I started to enjoy food, love the gym and feel energized like never before.

HARD WORK

This is where the honest truths are laid bare. I will be the first to admit that my journey wasn't a breeze, as I'm sure those of you who've dabbled with diets will know. There were times when all I wanted was to stay in bed and eat ice cream and the idea of even stepping one foot in the gym filled me with dread. But I couldn't allow myself to return to the disordered and unhealthy way of living that I had worked so hard to move away from.

What it required was the understanding that I needed to make change, the commitment and consistency to see it through and the knowledge that this was now my normal, and I wouldn't return to bad habits ever again.

I needed to make change, the commitment and consistency to see it through and the knowledge that this was now my normal.

Alice x

HOW IT ALL BEGAN

Being healthy can sound scary and complicated – it isn't. It is about being realistic and consistent and this book will show you how.

We all form food-related opinions and patterns from a very young age and they can be hard to break. It is all about educating yourself and the first thing to learn is that there is no such thing as a quick fix that gives you a result for life.

We all have different relationships with nutrition and food and I am happy to share mine here to show you how I got started on this clean eating path. Looking back I can see that my thoughts about food weren't always straightforward. From a young age there had always been triggers that would set me off on a period of binge eating that I couldn't control. I was a classic example of someone who struggled every day to overcome my bad eating habits. I would repeatedly fall off the diet wagon, only to climb back on, dispirited by failure and even more desperate to shift the weight. It became a destructive, depressing cycle I was locked into. I now know this is so common. We feel like failures and don't know how to change things in a permanent way; so we just carry on doing the same thing and feeling bad. I had tried every diet out there, particularly the quick-fix 'goal' diets designed to shed the pounds as quickly as possible. The problem was that I would never quite banish the 7lb the diet books promised, and then I would watch as the few pounds I had shifted crept right back on. It felt like a constant war.

They say that eating habits are formed in childhood and I suppose in my case that is true. Growing up we would all sit down to a meal as a family. My mum liked cooking and there was always a delicious range of food that all kids like, sometimes healthy and sometimes less so, but always home cooked and fresh. We didn't eat McDonald's or pizza (I didn't taste my first Big Mac until I went to university!) but my mum always served a pudding after every meal and that was very much the norm, even if we weren't particularly hungry after our main meal. It was just our family routine.

Looking back I suppose there were two things that had a lasting impact on how I interpreted food and nutrition. One was that my mum was very overweight when I was young and the other was that my sister was diagnosed with Type 1 diabetes when she was 12. In my mind the two things were very linked, in that it was only after my sister's diagnosis that my mum decided to tackle her weight and rather than turn to a programme or club, she was determined to do it herself. She did so well, changing what she ate and upping her exercise output. She lost a lot of weight and worked hard to change some of her attitudes and habits around food and mealtimes. It was a real turning point for the whole family and she has never looked back.

My sister's diabetes is hereditary on my dad's side. As a child we had watched our grandfather live with it and it was tough as he was poorly for a lot of my childhood, so hearing my sister had the same thing was scary. It became a firm turning point for my mum – things had to change on the food front in a very definite way. It was a medical need not a lifestyle one and it meant rethinking even the small things and overhauling what was in the fridge. It was actually the tiny changes I noticed first. Suddenly there wasn't any fruit juice in the door of the fridge, and we were encouraged to snack on fresh fruit instead of the cupboards full of crisps and biscuits. My mum became very interested in nutrition and started reading lots and experimenting with new recipes.

Before my sister's diagnosis we had a routine when it came to sweet treats. When we weren't at school, we would be given a daily allowance of sweets in a cup. It was up to us if we ate them all in one go or saved them for throughout the day, but they were there. And then suddenly they weren't. My parents didn't make a big deal of it or try and scare us with a big 'chat', but we knew why these changes were being made and obviously my sister has grown up having to manage it herself. She learned from a young age to adopt a balanced approach to what she drank and ate and found her way through to a manageable place.

It does not matter how slowly you go as long as you do not stop.

So suddenly, we were all much more focused on healthy foods, food that were good or bad for my sister and foods that would help my mum keep the weight off. It was a real change to the household, but in a way that felt very natural. It wasn't really this that had the big impact on me. The real change in my approach and attitude to food came when I went to Sixth Form College. I suppose it is the same for a lot of teenagers, body comparison became more apparent a lot of my friends ate what they wanted and were naturally very slim. But I also went through some tricky times and I began to find comfort in food. Having learned more about this since starting my Instagram page, I know that some people stop eating completely when they are stressed and some find comfort from feeling full. I was certainly in the second camp.

When it came to eating, I used to restrain myself in front of people, desperately trying to portray the image that I ate well and watched my weight, that I was 'good' about food. I'd eat things like Special K and would endlessly snack on Müller Light yoghurt and cereal bars, believing they were healthy. On the outside I looked in control and like I knew how to feed my body well, and then I would go off and binge eat on everything and anything when I got home. I would eat until I felt uncomfortably full and sick.

It was this incredibly disordered eating pattern that was then exacerbated when I went away to university because I didn't deal with it. Being accepted into the Bird College of Dance, Music and Theatre Performance was a dream come true. I thought I could 'out dance' my bad eating habits, given I was doing a degree that involved dancing practically all day, but the opposite turned out to be true. I just didn't understand that my whole attitude needed an overhaul.

Like most people who go away, I found university a real adjustment. Sport and exercise generally hadn't played a huge part in my life growing up, though I had always absolutely loved dancing, and particularly ballet. I went to classes three times a week and dreamed of being a ballerina when I grew up. Sadly, however, it wasn't long before I realized that I just wasn't built to be a ballet dancer – I wasn't long and lean, I was short and slightly round, and I remember being jealous of some of the more lithe girls in my class. It is a hard lesson to learn that genetics and physicality play a large part in determining dreams and maybe that is something I carried forward into later life. Either way, it only helped enhance my determination to find something else I could fully commit to. I wanted to uncover the right thing and excel.

THE GREATEST PLEASURE IN LIFE IS DOING WHAT PEOPLE SAY YOU CAN'T DO

The physically demanding nature of my degree was the first time I entertained the idea that I needed to make some changes. In terms of sports, I had enjoyed PE at school but never really excelled at any particular sport. At secondary school my friends were all in the 'sporty' crowd, all playing lacrosse and netball for the A teams, whilst I took more of an interest in drama and performing arts.

I remember absolutely dreading games lessons and always trying to forge notes to feign injury so I could get out of it!! My family were never that into exercise either. My mum, like me, would attempt all sorts of things to try and lose weight, from expensive personal trainers to tennis lessons, but nothing that she found seemed to work. My dad played the odd bit of golf or cricket, but was never really that mad about anything in particular.

The first year away at university passed in a bit of blur – though one of the things that stood out early on was the fact I had to cook for myself. This was something that I'd never really done before and I was really hopeless! As a result I turned to comfort food and simple, quick meals that would fill a void, but were far from nourishing. I just carried on eating rubbish and filling my body with unhealthy 'fuel'. It was in the dance studio though where I began to suffer the most. I was riddled with insecurity about my body and my confidence was at an all-time low, I was suffering with bad skin and excruciating fatigue. By the time I got to the end of my first year, I felt hopeless. I'd worked so hard to get there, I adored being on stage and it felt like I had found the thing I loved, but I hated the way I looked and was in terrible shape, so standing in front of a full-length mirror every day, unflattering leotards and all, wasn't the best idea. In truth, despite dancing for eight solid hours a day, I was putting on weight. It must be a bit like signing up to *Strictly Come Dancing* because you want to shed some pounds but then getting bigger. The truth is that you will only lose weight if you pay as much attention to what you eat and use to fuel your body. It is as much about input as it is output and if they aren't in tandem, you won't see results.

I felt so low in confidence and spent my time constantly comparing myself to others. Everywhere I looked there was someone prettier and thinner. How could I be doing so much exercise and getting bigger? I knew it was bad, but I didn't know how to fix it. It is funny really as I think back. Getting accepted to the Bird College was such a special moment, and yet all I can remember about that time were friends excitedly telling me that I was bound to 'lose loads of weight' as I would be 'dancing for hours every single day'. One particular friend was so excited for me, but she didn't congratulate me for all my hard work, instead she said, 'It is amazing, you will NEVER have to diet again.'

The opposite was true and the crunch came when I received my end-of-first-year report. I was devastated. Every single note commented that I lacked the physical strength and the confidence to be a star performer.

It was awful, but I knew, as I started my second term I had to take control. It was the first moment I realized that only I was in charge of what I put into my body and that I would get out exactly what I put in. Fuelling myself with junk wasn't going to help me. I was relying on my body, but treating it terribly. A shutter came down and I realized I needed, and wanted, to feel healthy and good about myself.

I began the 'clean eating' experimentation tentatively. After all, my whole life had been spent eating erratically, establishing bad habits and not understanding the impact that would have on my mood. But the shift was immediate, even with just the smallest tweaks to my everyday life. Like most people I didn't have the first idea where to begin, so I started looking online at what others were doing to eat healthily and lose weight.

It is important to make clear that at this early stage, and for the first time, I knew I needed to feel good as well as look good. To do well in my degree I needed strength, confidence and self-belief and bad food wasn't going to give me that. I needed to eat food that improved my energy levels, helped me manage my weight and gave me mental strength too. It wasn't about diets and calorie counting, it was about taking control and nurturing my body with nourishment.

I began to understand that food could be seen as medicine to make my body feel better, not something to be stuffed down because I was hungry, or something to be eaten guiltily because I felt sad about something or didn't like what I saw in the mirror. I gave myself a few ground rules about food:

1. It always needed to taste delicious
2. It must not be tricky to make
3. It mustn't involve expensive or obscure ingredients (I was a student after all)
4. I wouldn't cook it just because it was 'healthy'

Once I had a handle on the basics, I started putting my own spin on things. I decided that I had a better chance of sticking to a new regime if I made small changes. The first thing I looked at was the food I ate for breakfast – the meal we

A fit, healthy body – that's the best fashion statement

are brought up to believe 'sets us up for the day'. It seems so obvious, but our mood is bound to be dictated by what we put into our bodies, especially at the start of the day. Out went the sugary cereal (fortified and devoid of most original nutrients to extend its shelf life) and in came the fresh eggs.

I experimented with various foods and started to understand more, but it felt very isolating and I wanted to learn more and reach out to others with what I was doing, so that's when I decided to post my recipes online. It was definitely the combination of making the food and then posting it publicly that motivated me to make an effort, both with ingredients and the presentation. The truth is that if something looks beautiful on the plate, you are more likely to enjoy eating it.

My approach isn't scientific or rule-bound, it is relaxed and based on combining ingredients I like and that will provide me with the energy and fuel I needed to really push myself. This was first a priority in my dancing for my degree, then in my gym workouts and now on stage in my theatre job. It is about identifying the factors that underpin your current relationship with food, understanding the emotion behind it and retraining yourself so that you feel informed and strong.

The main push came from the fact that I immediately began to see results. I started sleeping better, my moods evened out and my skin cleared up. I felt good and like I could tackle anything.

It was then that the exercise came in. Given that I was dancing all day, you'd have thought that once I'd changed my diet, that would have been enough. But that was the first rule I learned – not all exercise is good exercise and you can't out-train a bad diet. You can spend an hour wandering around the gym, using the machines badly, and achieve nothing for your body. Twenty minutes can be all you need – if you do it right.

It has changed my life and it will change yours too.

I turned back to the internet and found help and hints that allowed me to construct my own bespoke exercise regime, in my case with the help of LDN Muscle. The key is consistency and sticking to a plan – that way every area sees an improvement. But I do have rest days – and you should too.

Clean eating has been well documented and interpreted in a whole host of ways, but to me it is simple. Clean eating meant cutting all the rubbish from my diet, binning the foods that made me fall on the sofa exhausted, not because of my job or my college course, but because the food I was eating was bad for me. Deciding to do this quite literally forced me to realign my relationship with food, to stop using it as my crutch and to start understanding the impact it had on me. It was about listening to my body and making long-term changes.

Everyone has a different path. This book isn't going to dictate anything to you – there is no one-size-fits-all when it comes to food and wellbeing. That's why this book isn't a diet, it is a way of life. There are other books on the market that promise a quick fix, but the truth is that unless you make a change for life, those books will always bring you back to needing a book like this.

It has taken me a long time to get to the point where I feel I want to share my thoughts with you and my only hope is that this book makes you more mindful about the food you choose and about incorporating some kind of exercise into your life. We have to understand that the food we eat has a direct effect on how we feel. This knowledge has changed my life, and it will change yours too.

This book will help you achieve health and happiness, no matter what size you are. My recipes aren't for people who have hours a day free to spend in the gym. This is a book for busy people who want to look and feel great.

It felt like a big deal when I first started. We all have factors that come into play when we select the food choices we do, and I needed to think about what they were and why I made them. Everyone has their own backstory and this book is mine. Yours will be different, but I hope that this will help show you it is possible to make changes that last for life.

You have just got to want it and once you are sure you do, this book will help you get it!

FREQUENTLY ASKED QUESTIONS

How often do you exercise?

I exercise between four and five times a week. Each session is about an hour long, allowing time for a proper warm up and a cool down period. However, I always believe in listening to my body, so this is not a strict regime. If I am tired or sore I will always make sure I rest and won't force myself to the gym.

Do you have rest days?

No matter how quickly you want to see results, the body should have rest days to allow the muscles to recover. This will enable you to sustain your programme without injury. In the recipe section there is a selection of lunches and dinners specifically created for non-exercise days – these are lighter and slightly lower in calories.

How long did your transformation take?

My transformation took me about a year. That said, I am still always learning and adjusting my diet. It is a work in progress as I learn more about how my body responds to different foods and exercise.

Do you ever have cheat meals?

I have totally changed my approach to eating since beginning my journey. I have fallen in love with making, eating and enjoying good, whole nutritious foods, and so have found that I crave sugary sweet treats and 'junk' foods less. That being said, I still do sometimes crave my favourite foods like ice cream, pastries and cereal, to name a few, and will usually cheat with things like this once a week, usually on a Sunday evening. I also just eat mindfully. If I'm going out for dinner with friends, I don't want to be antisocial and scrutinize the menu looking for something 'clean'. I will simply have a lighter lunch or breakfast, make sure I hit the gym and then enjoy exactly what I want for dinner, and not feel any guilt at all.

What do you snack on?

I have lots of different snacks that I alternate between during the week. I like to always have some hard-boiled eggs, which I'll prep on a Sunday evening, stored in the fridge to grab for a quick protein hit, as well as chopped vegetables and dips for light snacking. Rice cakes, cashew nuts and fruit are also some of my favourite quick snacks. My all time favourite snack has to be Greek yogurt with fruit and crushed nuts – a delicious hit of protein, fats and carbs and it tastes delicious too!

Do you drink alcohol?

I have never been a big drinker so I'd be lying if I said this was a huge change I've made, but I do now make different choices when it comes to drinking. If I'm heading out with friends, I absolutely love a glass of Champagne and will have one or two, or sometimes spirits like a vodka and slimline tonic.

THE PROMISE

WHAT?

I have heard from, and spoken to, so many people who constantly tell me that they struggle to lose weight, that they're unhappy with their bodies, and that diets just don't seem to be working for them. No matter what they do, the weight doesn't shift, they feel miserable and so they eat more – and so the cycle continues.

It was with this in mind that I wanted to create this book, to dispel all the diet myths and prove that achieving your desired physique doesn't have to involve you taking drastic measures for a short period of time, only to then see the weight creep back on.

The Body Bible will provide you with delicious, easy to make recipes and straightforward workouts that will help you create and maintain a lean and healthy body; you will never have to look at, or think about, a diet again.

We all want to be able to enjoy food, to feel fabulous and to live long, happy, healthy lives – that should be our main goal. However, placing stress upon the body by following a diet that promotes an extreme reduction in calories just isn't the solution. What this book will provide you with is not only the tools to help you achieve your end goal, but also a flexible and sustainable way of eating that doesn't just last for a few weeks. These recipes can be created again and again, and have taste and flavour at their core, while also being balanced and nutrient-dense to ensure you aren't left feeling hungry.

HOW?

It's important to explain how I will help you achieve this. Losing weight can, for most people, be simplified as an equation: calories in vs calories out. If you consume more calories than you are burning in a day, you will gain weight. If you consume fewer calories than you burn in a day, you will lose weight. With this in mind, it is my objective to help you enter into a realistic caloric deficit through nutrition and exercise in order for you to be able to lose weight. Following the recipes in the first half of this book and building in 4 or 5 workouts a week into your routine, will ensure you lose weight and develop lean muscle definition. This will be be achieved by targeting specific areas of your body. You need long-term commitment dedicated to both areas of the book. It has become a way of life for me now, and having lost the desired amount of weight, I continue to maintain this way of life.

The recipes in this book are all designed to help you eat a balance of nutritious foods, meaning you won't feel as though you are dieting at all. Having said this, it is important to be mindful of calorie intake while not obsessing over it. For example, we all know avocados are good for us, but we must also remember that they are calorie dense, so eating five a day will take you well over your recommended daily calorie intake – this means you will gain weight. I like to have rough ideas of how much I am consuming at each meal so that I can keep track of how much I am eating on a given day. It's important that your calorie intake is specific and individual to you and focuses less on what other people are doing. We all live very different lives, with different activity levels, so naturally our calorie intake is going to be totally unique. For example, I am 5ft 1in, weigh around 8 stone and consume about 1,800 calories per day, but this can fluctuate depending on my activity levels.

While actively consuming less, we can also create a deficit through burning calories during exercise. The exercises within this book are created to help you have a structured programme to be used alongside the recipes. The workouts are designed to be completed at home, or in the garden, and so, unfortunately, excuses just don't cut it! Getting active is so essential to looking and feeling good, and these workouts are designed to help you gain confidence with body weight exercises that you can then put into practise in the gym, or continue to perfect at home. The truth is that simply eating the food I suggest isn't enough – the definition and strength of my body were achieved with exercise, and lots of it. There really is no pain without gain! It is essential you understand that both elements have been so vital to the change in my body and my mind.

WHY?

We live in a world where there are fast food restaurants on every high street, where obesity is an epidemic, and where exercise seems to have been lost in favour of computer games and electronic devices. It might sound like I'm being a little dramatic here, but making a decision to change your lifestyle, deciding to create healthy habits and develop a knowledge and understanding of what constitutes a healthy, balanced diet, will ensure that you don't become another statistic. It is the best decision I ever made and this book will set you on the path I am so grateful to be taking.

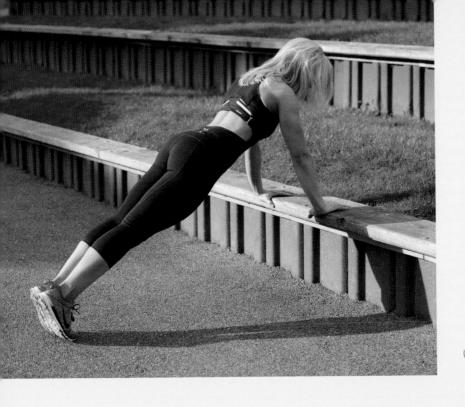

The workouts are designed to be completed at home, or in the garden, and so, unfortunately, excuses just don't cut it!

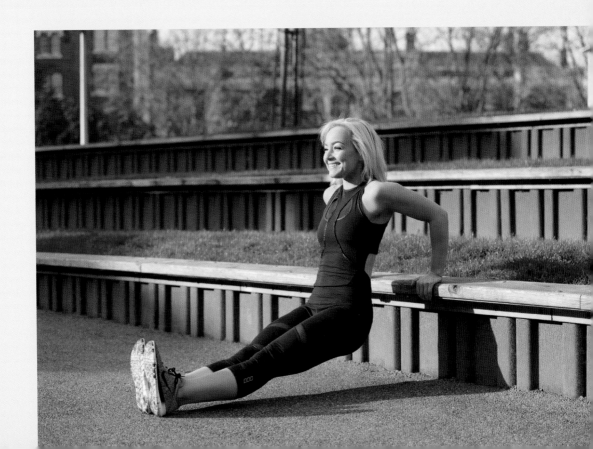

What the book IS

A guaranteed path to a healthy mind and healthy body

A lifestyle you can live on a budget – everything you need can be bought from your local supermarket – no need to step inside a health food shop for expensive supplements!

A way to take control of your mind and body

A regime that will give you more energy, help you sleep and, vitally, help you lose weight

A book that will empower and energise you to make a permanent change

A winning combination of healthy eating and exercise that you will love

A promise of permanent results

A collection of delicious, non-fussy, stress-free recipes for busy people – both on excercise and rest days

A group of exercises that target specific body areas and issues, such as abs, and that can be done anywhere

What the book ISN'T

A yo-yo diet

About restriction or denial

About being hard on yourself

About cutting out specific food groups

About feeling hungry

Hints and tips before you get started

This book is not a diet; it is a way of life.

It will teach you to love food that's good for you, as well as developing a relationship with food that enables you to break free from the restrictions of dieting. Food is fuel, it's what keeps us alive and it should be enjoyed, not feared. It's with this in mind that I've shared these recipes, which I hope will help you to achieve a healthy mind and body.

Flexibility is essential.

A balanced approach is what helps keep you focused and on track.

This book is all about ease and simplicity but isn't

just aimed at fat loss. It's for people who want to feel good from the inside out. Nutrition affects all aspects of our daily existence, and taking steps to educate yourself about fitness, nutrition, health and wellbeing with this book, no matter what your end goals are, is going to benefit you.

NEW MONDAY, NEW WEEK, NEW GOALS

Drink up! The body is made of about 60 per cent water, and keeping hydrated is essential for you to function and feel your best. My advice: carry water with you always, and aim to drink no less than two litres of water a day, and more if you're exercising.

Sugar. It's a hot topic at the moment, and a real bone of contention. Be aware of sugar content in foods – you'd be surprised how much some everyday products contain, and it can hinder fat loss. Don't obsess over it, but checking labels of things like chopped tomatoes and sauces can help you make better choices.

Should I go wheat or gluten free?

I believe that unless you have a diagnosed medical condition, you shouldn't stress about eliminating these from your diet completely. My approach to eating is to consume mainly whole nutrient-dense foods. So, with the recipes that follow, we can begin to re-establish a healthy digestive system. This means your system will be free from heavily processed foods that lack the ability to nourish and power our bodies properly.

I am absolutely passionate about the taste, flavour, texture and colour of food
and believe that eating should be an experience we enjoy. All my recipes can be tailored to your tastes and goals – be it by adding or reducing carbs within a dish, swapping salmon for a preferred fish, or if you don't like squash, use sweet potato. The beauty of them is their ability to be adapted to each individual's needs without compromising on flavour.

Fats should not be feared! They are a great source of energy and provide vital nutrients for the body. With fats being the most calorie dense of all the macronutrients we should be slightly mindful when consuming them - for example eating five avocados a day, or a whole bag of nuts, would provide a whopping amount of calories, but in moderation they are, in my opinion, an absolutely essential part of your diet.

Alcohol. There is no getting away from it - alcohol has very little nutritional value. If you are trying to lose weight, the truth is that wine and beer will be your enemy. Not only does alcohol slow down the weight loss process, but it is loaded with sugar, which can stop the body from burning fat. This obviously means it will hinder you shedding the pounds. Drinking lots also stops the body functioning at full capacity the next day - you eat more sugary and carb-heavy foods and feel less like exercise.

Tips:
· If you are a big drinker, try saving yourself for one day of drinking a week.
· Match each alcoholic drink with a glass of water.

However, my approach in this book is that, with the right balance, we can achieve both a healthy mind and body, so consuming alcohol on occasion is fine.

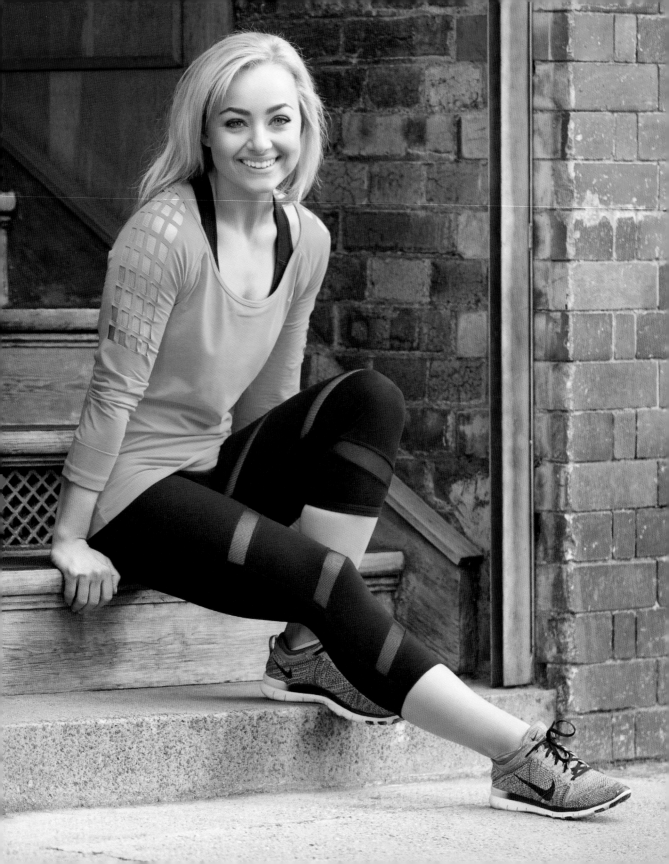

GETTING STARTED

There are ways of making all your favourite foods healthy – it is just a question of learning how. I am not a chef, but a cook in my own home. I love experimenting with flavour and texture. Healthy doesn't equal boring! The book is full of tips, and quick, simple weekday recipes, plus an area-specific exercise programme, complete with advice on when to schedule rest days. This is a lifestyle choice, not a short-term fix. I promise you it is worth it.

Do:

- Make small changes first
- Learn and understand the value of calories
- Prepare recipes in advance
- Celebrate food that makes you feel great and that you enjoy making
- Remember – you can't out-train a bad diet
- Find exercise you love – it is vital

Don't:

- Worry – the recipes are not expensive
- Blame a hectic lifestyle for eating badly
- Feel like you're on a diet
- Be too hard on yourself. Deciding to make a change is the first step

Example of a day of simple swaps:

BEFORE (STARTING WEIGHT OF 9.5 STONES):

BREAKFAST:
Two slices of toast with butter and jam
SNACK: Sugary cereal bars
LUNCH:
Jacket potato with tuna, baked beans and cheese
SNACK:
Coffee and biscuits
DINNER:
Spaghetti bolognese and lots of cheese
DESSERT:
An apple, a few biscuits and small chocolate bars

AFTER (CURRENT WEIGHT OF 8 STONES):

BREAKFAST:
One slice of rye bread, toasted, with scrambled eggs
SNACK:
Two rice cakes with peanut butter
LUNCH:
Peri-peri spiced chicken breast with butternut squash and broccoli
SNACK:
Homemade banana muffin with blueberries
DINNER:
Grilled turkey breast with warm lentil, feta and tomato salad and sautéed kale
DESSERT:
Greek yogurt with raspberries and two squares of dark chocolate

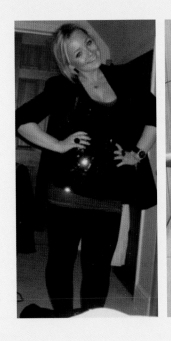

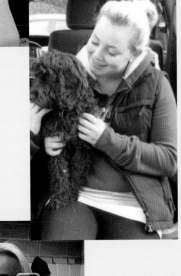

A simple change is all you need

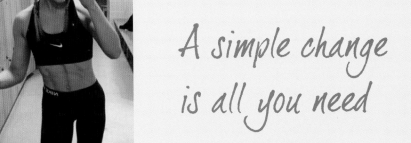

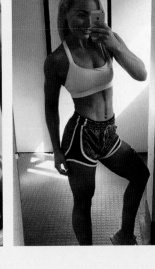

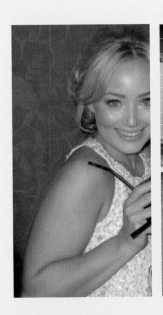

Green and Lean. We all know we should eat our greens. Including leafy, fibrous vegetables in our diet aids and improves digestion, and provides essential micronutrients to our diet like iron and calcium, and they are also high in antioxidants. Examples of these are spinach, kale, cabbage and broccoli.

Why Coconut Oil. Coconut oil is my preferred choice of cooking oil because of its high smoke point. Unlike other oils like vegetable or olive oil, it is less damaged and chemically altered when heated, and doesn't denature, therefore making it arguably the healthiest oil to cook with.

Mad About Avocados. As well as tasting absolutely delicious, avocados are also extremely good for you, providing vitamin E, potassium and iron, and a plentiful source of good monounsaturated fats.

Fats: what and why? The four main types of fat found in our diet are: monounsaturated fats, polyunsaturated fats, saturated fats and trans fats. Unsaturated fats (mono and poly) are often the fats associated with the label 'healthy fats' and foods that fall into this category are things like avocados, nuts, peanut butter, oily fish and unsaturated oils. These are loaded with nutrients and will nourish your body whilst also keeping you satiated. The one we really need to be careful of and avoid at all costs is artificial trans fats, which can be found in things like margarine, chips and fast food, as these can contribute to cancer, heart disease and diabetes.

Herbal and Fruit Teas. If you are suffering from sweet cravings, try a warm fruit or herbal tea instead of reaching for sugar-loaded snacks. My favourites are peppermint, raspberry and strawberry.

Protein has been shown to be 25-30 per cent more satiating than any of the other food groups and is therefore essential to keeping you fuller for longer. Including lean meats like chicken and fish in your diet will help you avoid feeling hungry.

HAPPY AS
LONG AS
I'M NOT
HUNGRY

Cupboard essentials

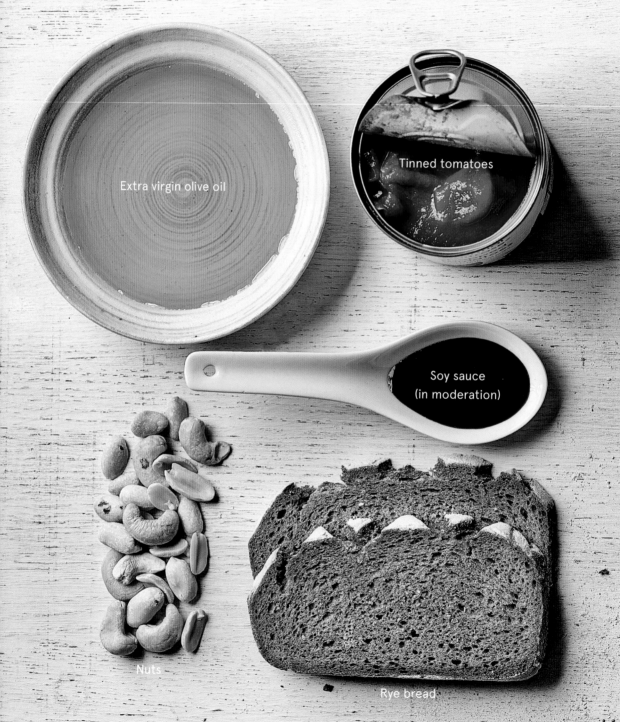

Extra virgin olive oil

Tinned tomatoes

Soy sauce
(in moderation)

Nuts

Rye bread

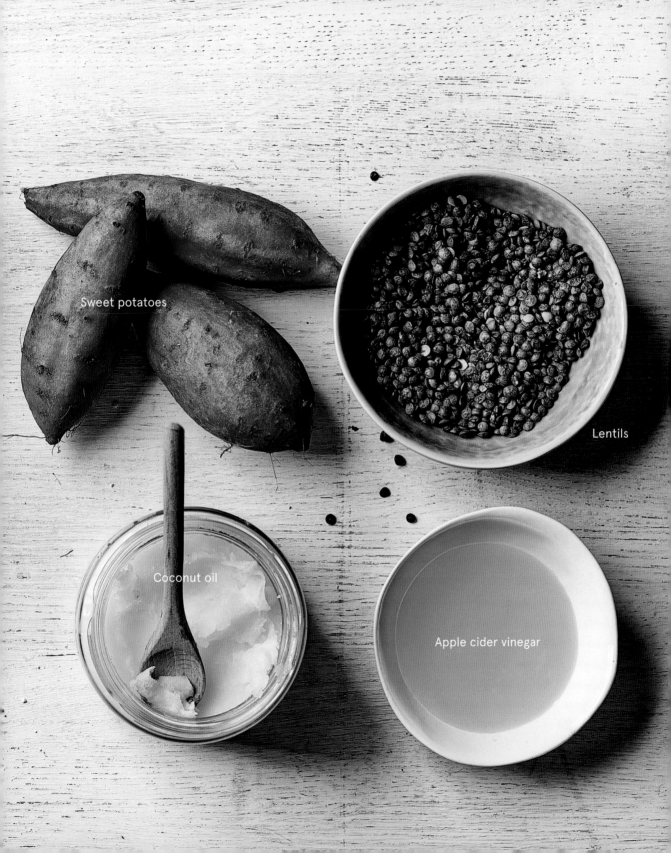

Sweet potatoes

Lentils

Coconut oil

Apple cider vinegar

Fresh essentials

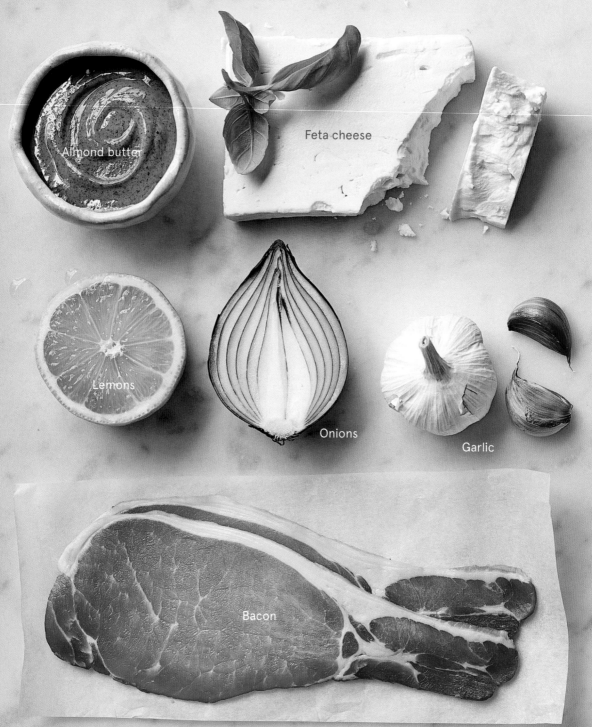

Almond butter

Feta cheese

Lemons

Onions

Garlic

Bacon

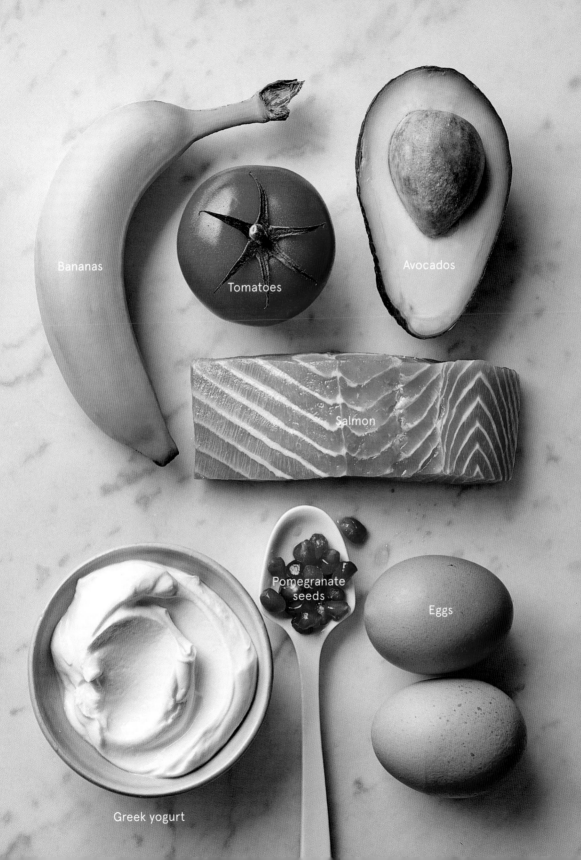

Bananas

Tomatoes

Avocados

Salmon

Pomegranate
seeds

Eggs

Greek yogurt

Seasoning essentials

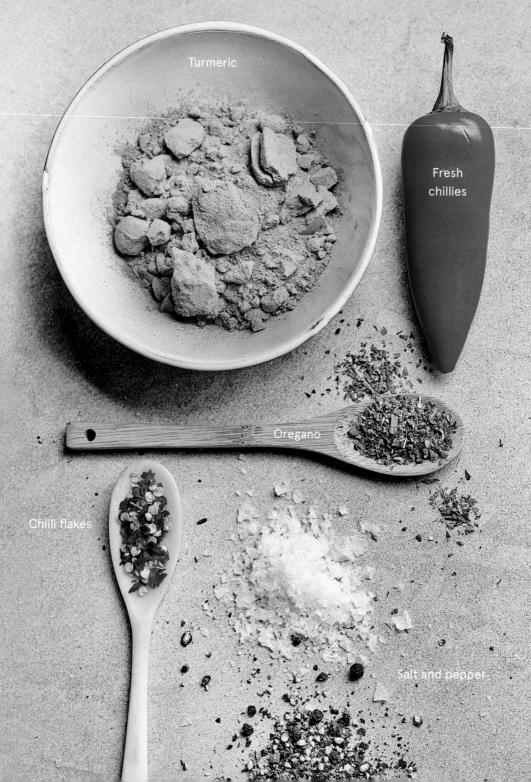

Turmeric

Fresh chillies

Oregano

Chilli flakes

Salt and pepper

Garlic powder

Lime juice

Cumin seeds

Cayenne pepper

Cinnamon

Paprika

FOOD

Food is our fuel. It's how we function day to day and it keeps us alive. It's social, it's delicious and how we consume it has a direct impact on our ability to lose fat.

There is a common belief that the ideal fat-loss equation is 80 per cent diet and 20 per cent exercise and I agree wholeheartedly with that. Despite exercising more than the average person throughout my Theatre Performance degree, it was only when I made changes to my diet that I noticed a real difference to my physique. With just a little education on how better to fuel your body, you can look and feel completely different. Most importantly, these changes can be sustained for longer than the typical 'six-week cleanse' – they can be for life.

I'm going to be clear with you here – this book isn't going to be a miserable low-calorie liquid detox, or involve you throwing away 90 per cent of the contents of your fridge and cupboards and heading to the most obscure aisle of your local health-food shop. My aim is to help you to discover an achievable, sustainable way of eating that will nourish and fuel your body. This book will change your perception of how to eat and help you to achieve and maintain your desired physique. There is no quick fix, but if you commit and work hard, like me, you will have a happy mind and the body you've always wanted.

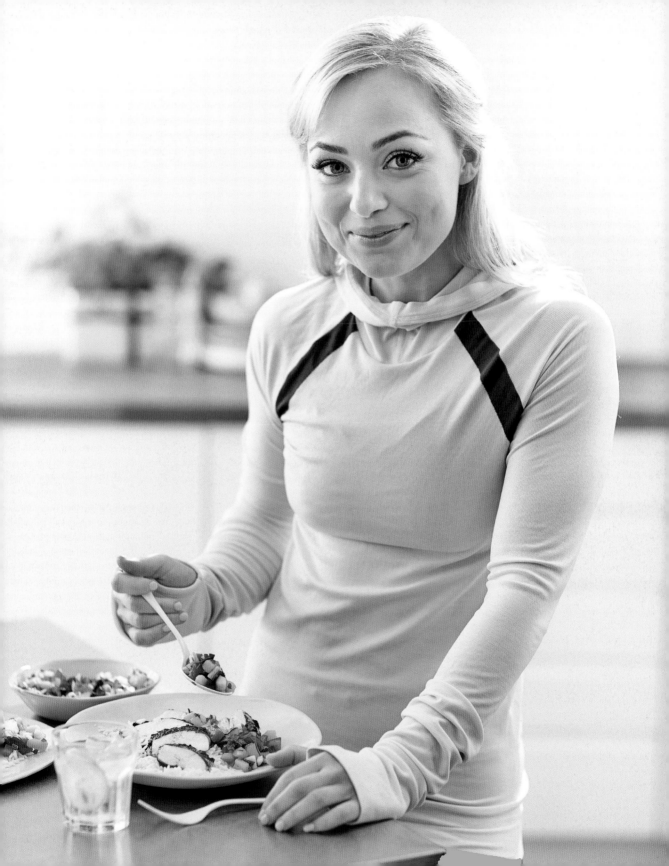

BREAKFAST

For me, breakfast is the most important meal of the day. When you wake, your body has been fasting since your dinner the previous evening, so it is important to have a meal that will fill you up and provide you with the right balance of nutrients to tackle the day. The problem is, we've developed an unhealthy concept of what breakfast should consist of – sugary cereals, toast loaded with unhealthy toppings, even low-fat yogurt that is branded as 'healthy'. They all sound great, but really they aren't the best way to set you up for a busy day. Without going into too much 'science stuff', sugar-laden cereals and spreads can cause a spike in insulin levels, which leads to that horrible mid-morning energy crash where you want to eat everything in sight.

Simply switching up your breakfast will create a slower, more consistent release of energy throughout the morning and help you to avoid that mid-morning slump. Eating a breakfast high in protein will also help fill you up far more than any cereal or breakfast bar, meaning that you won't find yourself hungry and needing to snack on calorific foods throughout the morning.

Stuffed French Toast with Almond Butter and Banana

The sweet aroma of almond and banana is the ultimate treat. This is a luxurious and delicious breakfast and is a real weekend favourite for me.

2 slices of rye or wholegrain
    bread
2 tbsp almond butter
½ banana, thinly sliced
1 free-range egg
½ tsp ground cinnamon
50ml unsweetened almond milk
coconut oil, for frying
fresh berries and Greek
    yogurt, to serve (optional)

SERVES 1

1. Slice the bread into halves and layer up the bottom halves with your almond butter and banana slices, then sandwich together with the top half.

2. In a shallow dish, whisk together the egg, cinnamon and almond milk until fully combined, then soak both sides of your sandwiches until well coated and moist.

3. Heat a little coconut oil in a non-stick frying pan then gently lay your sandwiches in to fry for about 4 minutes on each side.

4. Plate up and top with fresh berries and a tablespoon of Greek yogurt, if you like.

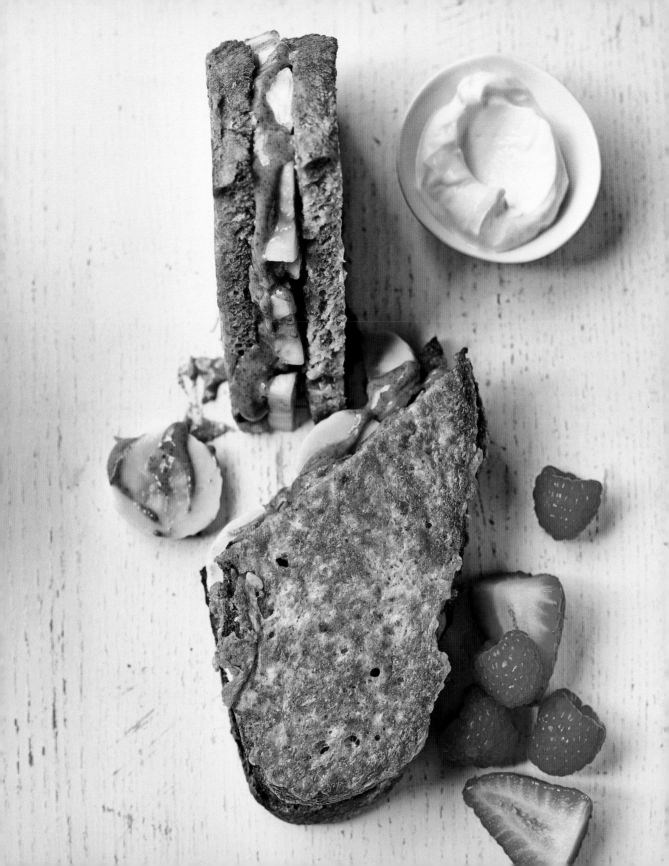

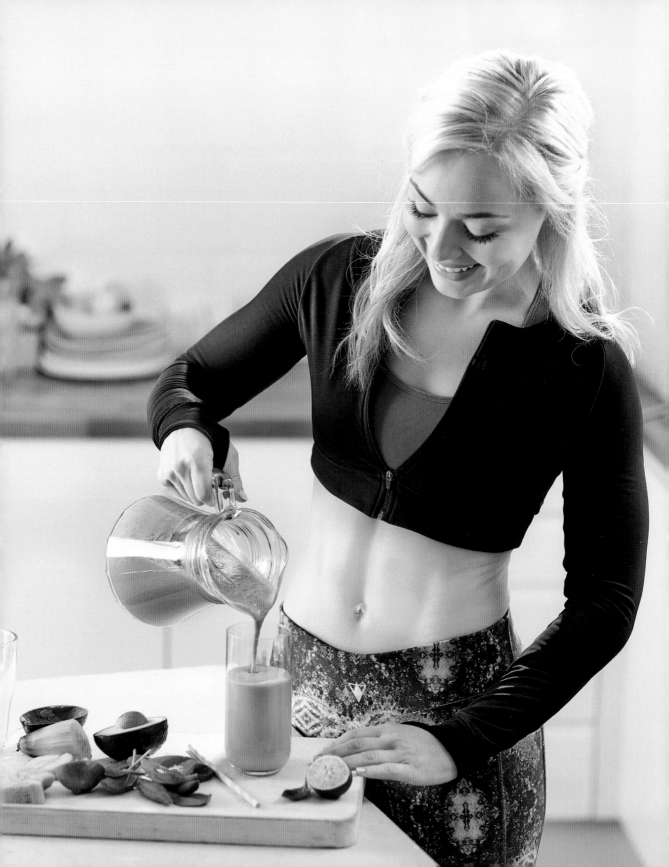

Super-green Breakfast Smoothie

If you struggle to get your greens in, this is a quick and simple idea that combines both savoury and sweet in a delicious smoothie packed full of protein and antioxidants.

1 large kiwi, peeled and cut into chunks

½ ripe avocado, stone removed and flesh cut into chunks

1 tbsp Greek yogurt

1 handful of fresh spinach

juice of 1 lime

¼ cucumber, peeled and cut into chunks

100ml unsweetened almond milk

SERVES 2

Blitz all the ingredients in a blender until smooth and serve.

Coconut and Vanilla Protein Pancakes with Mango Chia Seed Jam

Who doesn't love pancakes? Enjoy these topped with a sweet and light chia seed jam for a protein hit to satisfy that sweet tooth without the added sugar!

FOR THE JAM

50g fresh mango

1 tsp desiccated coconut

1 tsp chia seeds

100ml liquid egg white

1 scoop of vanilla whey
    protein powder
    (or preferred flavour)

½ tbsp ground flaxseed

½ banana, mashed

1 tsp desiccated coconut,
    plus extra to serve
    (optional)

coconut oil, for frying

SERVES 2

1. To make the jam, blitz the mango in a food processor until it is puréed. Add the coconut and chia seeds and blitz again briefly. Remove, place in a jar and leave to let the chia seeds absorb the liquid for a few minutes.

2. In a mixing bowl, whisk together the liquid egg white, protein powder and flaxseed. Once this is all combined, stir through the mashed banana and coconut.

3. Heat a small amount of coconut oil in a non-stick frying pan and set over a medium heat. Pour in about half of the pancake mixture and leave to cook until the bottom has set, then flip over to cook the other side. Repeat with the rest of the mixture.

4. To serve, plate up the pancakes and top with a good helping of jam and an extra sprinkling of desiccated coconut, if desired.

Banana and Fig Sweet Omelette

If you're not a savoury egg fan, try this sweet recipe with ripe figs and banana for a breakfast winner!

2 free-range eggs

1 banana, mashed

¼ tsp ground cinnamon, plus extra to dust (optional)

¼ tsp ground nutmeg

½ tsp coconut oil, for frying

2 fresh figs, cut into segments

SERVES 2

1. In a mixing bowl, whisk together the eggs and mashed banana until completely combined, then add the spices.

2. Preheat the grill.

3. Heat the coconut oil in a non-stick frying pan then pour in the banana and egg mixture.

4. Once the base has set, lay the fig segments onto the omelette and place the pan under the grill to cook the top.

5. Cut in half and serve with a light dusting of cinnamon, if desired.

Butternut Squash and Crispy Parma Ham Squeak with Fried Eggs

For breakfast, brunch or lunch, this combination packs in so much flavour while also being a great source of protein, fats and carbs.

250g butternut squash, peeled
    and cut into chunks
coconut oil, for frying
1 red onion, finely diced
2-3 slices of Parma ham, torn
    into small pieces
pinch of chilli flakes,
    plus extra for sprinkling
    (optional)
2 free-range eggs
sea salt and freshly ground
    black pepper

SERVES 1

1. Begin by bringing a saucepan of water to boil and add the butternut squash. Cook for 15 to 20 minutes until soft. Once cooked, drain and set aside to cool.

2. Heat a small amount of coconut oil in a frying pan and fry the red onion and Parma ham until the ham is crispy.

3. Transfer to a bowl, add the butternut squash and mash everything together with the chilli flakes and a good amount of seasoning.

4. Preheat the grill.

5. Heat a little more coconut oil in the pan and then add the squash mixture, flattening it down into a thick pancake shape. Cook until golden on the underside then place under the hot grill to cook the top.

6. Using a separate pan, fry the eggs until cooked.

7. Remove the butternut squash from the grill and allow to cool a little before sliding onto a plate and topping with the fried eggs.

8. Finish with an extra pinch of chilli flakes, if desired.

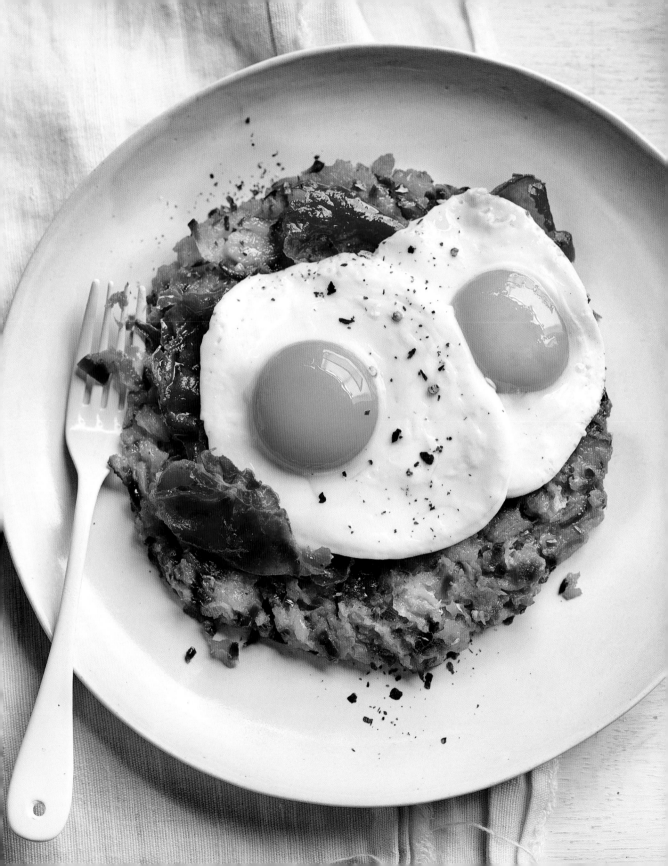

Deconstructed Breakfast Buttie

A healthy twist on an old favourite. Try this delicious alternative to your weekend greasy fry-up.

2-3 rashers of lean bacon

2 slices of rye bread

1 handful of rocket

1 large salad tomato, sliced

coconut oil, for frying

1 free-range egg

chilli flakes (optional)

sea salt and freshly ground black pepper

SERVES 1

1. Preheat the grill.

2. Place the bacon onto a foil-lined tray and put under the grill, removing halfway through to turn.

3. Meanwhile, toast the rye bread and then assemble on a plate with the rocket and tomato on top.

4. Heat a small amount of coconut oil in a pan and break the egg into the pan. Fry over a medium heat.

5. Once the bacon is cooked, remove from the grill and carefully assemble on top of the rocket and tomato, then top with the fried egg.

6. Season with a little salt and pepper, and chilli flakes, if desired.

Super-simple Tomato, Basil and Mozzarella Breakfast Omelette

This is a delicious twist on the good old-fashioned omelette and there is a real kick thanks to the sweet tomatoes and tangy basil. Ideal for hungry children, teenagers and mums and dads - a real family favourite!

2 large free-range eggs

coconut oil, for frying

1 handful of cherry
    tomatoes, halved

30-50g mozzarella

1 small handful of fresh
    basil leaves, torn

sea salt and freshly ground
    black pepper

SERVES 1

1. Preheat the grill.

2. Whisk the eggs and some salt and pepper until completely combined.

3. Heat the coconut oil in a non-stick frying pan, pour in the egg mixture, then scatter the tomatoes and mozzarella evenly over.

4. Once the base has cooked, remove from the hob and place under the grill to cook the top.

5. Once the top has cooked, plate up and serve with fresh basil leaves tossed evenly over.

Greek Yogurt with Caramelized Cinnamon Banana and Nectarine

Ideal for those of you who don't have much time in the mornings. This breakfast can be prepped in advance and enjoyed on the go!

200g Greek yogurt

coconut oil, for frying

1 banana, sliced

1 nectarine, stoned and cut
   into segments

ground cinnamon, to dust

1 tbsp almond butter

SERVES 1

1. Place the yogurt in a serving bowl.

2. Heat a small amount of coconut oil in a frying pan and add the fruit. Add a dusting of cinnamon until all the fruit is covered and leave to fry gently until slightly browned.

3. Remove from the heat and leave the fruit to stand for a few minutes before adding to the yogurt.

4. Top with the almond butter and an extra dusting of cinnamon, if desired.

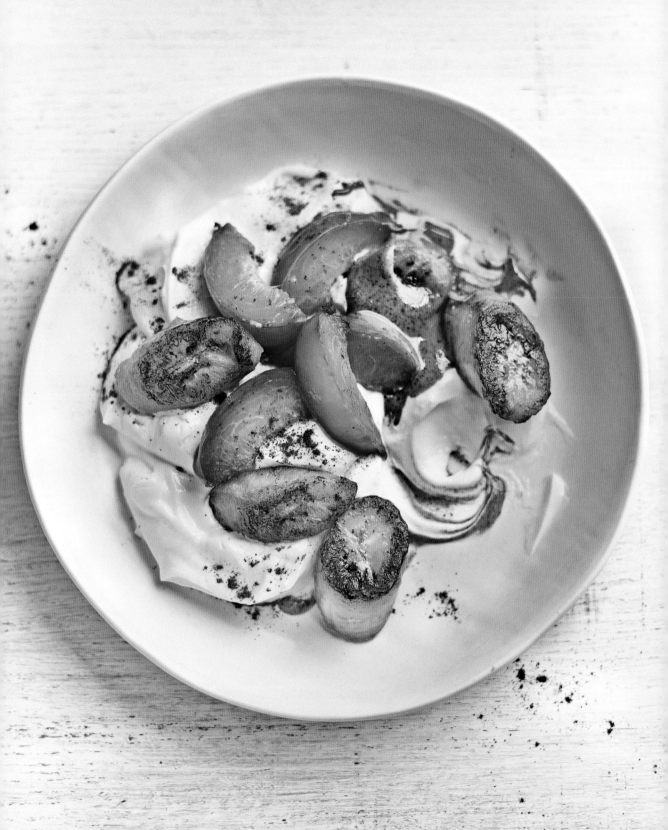

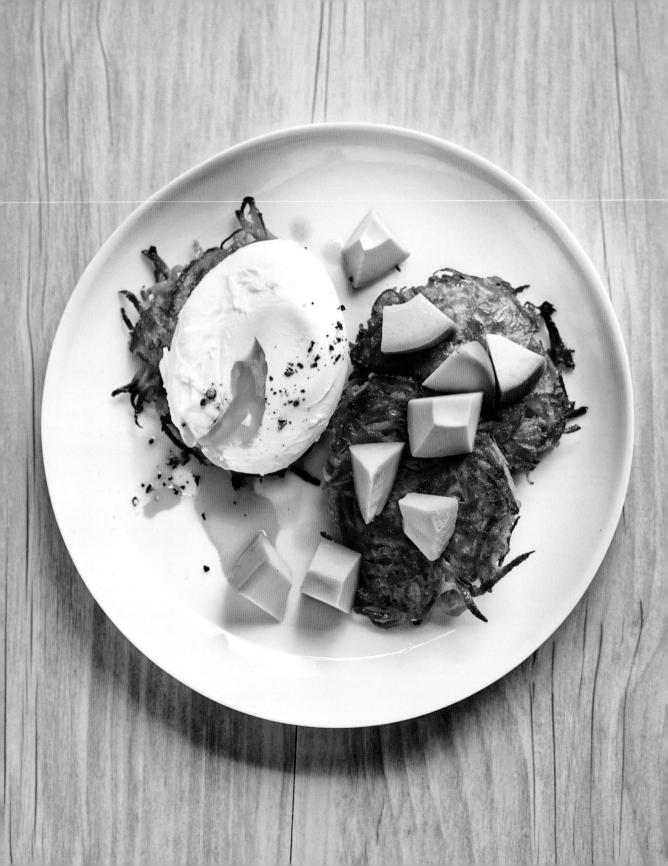

Sweet Potato Fritters with Poached Eggs and Avocado

A combination made in healthy-foodie heaven, this will be sure to satisfy you first thing in the morning!

2 small sweet potatoes, peeled and grated

3 free-range eggs

2 tsp coconut oil

1 tsp cider vinegar

½ ripe avocado, stone removed

sea salt and freshly ground black pepper

SERVES 2

1. Break one egg into a mixing bowl and whisk. Add the sweet potato, one teaspoon of the coconut oil and a good pinch of salt and pepper and mix until completely combined.

2. Using your hands, take a handful of the sweet potato mixture and form six palm-sized balls. Place in a hot frying pan with the remaining coconut oil, flattening gently as they cook to make a patty. Cook until golden then transfer to two plates.

3. Meanwhile, bring a large, wide pan of water with the cider vinegar to the boil. Turn the heat right down so it is very gently simmering and break the remaining eggs into the water to poach.

4. Leave to cook for about 3 minutes before removing with a slotted spoon to drain. Place on top of the sweet potato fritters.

5. Finally, cut the avocado into small chunks and assemble over the eggs and fritters.

Parsnip Chorizo Hash with Paprika and Fried Eggs

An amazing combination designed to help you think outside the cereal box. The tastes and textures in this dish are wonderful and it's a great one to share with the family!

coconut oil, for frying

2 red onions, finely diced

150g cooking chorizo, cut into small pieces

500g parsnips, grated

½ tsp smoked paprika

2 garlic cloves, crushed

4 free-range eggs

pinch of chilli flakes (optional)

sea salt and freshly ground black pepper

SERVES 2

1. Heat a small amount of coconut oil in a large frying pan and cook the red onion over a medium heat.

2. Add the chorizo to the pan, turn up the heat slightly and let this cook for a further 5 minutes.

3. Next, add the parsnips, paprika, garlic and a good pinch of salt and pepper and fry over a medium heat, stirring occasionally, until the parsnips are tender.

4. Make four individual spaces in the pan. Add a small amount of coconut oil to each of these before cracking the eggs into the centre of each one.

5. Once cooked, using a spoon, scoop each egg with the accompanying hash onto plates, topping with chilli flakes for an extra kick if desired.

Caramelized Banana and Peanut Butter Sundae

This is a proper sweet-treat start to the day and the ultimate perk-me-up breakfast for a hectic morning. The sundae can be put together the night before for an on-the-go nutritional breakfast.

1 banana, cut into chunks

ground cinnamon, to dust

2 tbsp rolled oats

coconut oil, for frying

200g Greek yogurt

2 tsp peanut butter

½ tsp agave nectar

SERVES 1

1. Begin by covering the banana with a light dusting of cinnamon.

2. Toast your oats in a dry frying pan for about a minute before removing from the heat and tipping into a bowl to cool slightly.

3. Heat a small amount of coconut oil in the hot pan then add the bananas and fry until they are slightly golden and crispy. Remove from the heat and leave to stand.

4. Mix the yogurt, peanut butter and agave nectar until well combined.

5. In a jar or dish, layer up half the yogurt, followed by half the oats and half of the banana slices. Repeat, finishing with a sprinkling more of cinnamon if desired.

The Healthy Foodie Favourite – Chilli-spiced Fried Egg and Smashed Avocado on Toasted Rye Bread

All your 'clean eating' staples on one plate, this dish is a real favourite of mine. You certainly don't start your day hungry, and the sprinkled chilli flakes mean it packs a punch first thing in the morning!

½ large ripe avocado

pinch of chilli flakes

coconut oil, for frying

1 free-range egg

1 slice of rye bread

sea salt

SERVES 1

1. On a chopping board, remove the stone and skin from the avocado and, using a fork, gently mash the flesh until smooth and season with a pinch of chilli flakes and sea salt.

2. In a frying pan, heat a small amount of coconut oil and break the egg in to fry.

3. Toast the rye bread, then spread with the mashed avocado.

4. Top with the fried egg and another pinch of chilli flakes, if desired.

A healthy outside starts from the inside

Warming Apple Crumble Porridge

Just right for those chilly winter mornings, this can be enjoyed first thing or post workout to replenish you and is a healthy twist on a much-loved dessert.

2 apples

coconut oil, for frying

1 tsp ground cinnamon

80g rolled oats

550ml unsweetened almond milk

¼ tsp ground nutmeg

20g jumbo oats

SERVES 2

1. Peel and core the apples, then dice them very finely.

2. In a frying pan, heat a small amount of coconut oil and fry the apples, covering them with a light dusting of cinnamon, until browned all over.

3. Next, in a non-stick pan, place the rolled oats, almond milk and nutmeg and bring to the boil. Stir often, then reduce the heat and leave to simmer for 3 to 4 minutes.

4. In a frying pan, dry fry the jumbo oats for 2 to 3 minutes until golden and crispy.

5. Serve the porridge in bowls and top with the apple and toasted oats.

Smoked Salmon and Scrambled Eggs

Incredibly simple and perfect for those with busy mornings and busy lives. This delivers on protein and essential omega-3 fatty acids to provide you with brain fuel for a busy day!

coconut oil, for frying

3 free-range eggs

1 tbsp whole milk

150g smoked salmon

½ tsp chopped fresh chives

150g cherry tomatoes, halved

1 small handful of pumpkin seeds

sea salt and freshly ground black pepper

SERVES 2

1. In a frying pan, heat a small amount of coconut oil and fry the tomatoes until slightly browned and soft, then transfer to a plate.

2. Whisk the eggs, milk and some salt and pepper together in a bowl.

3. Add another small amount of coconut oil to the frying pan, pour the eggs in, and stir often until they are scrambled. Plate up with the smoked salmon and top with fresh chives, tomatoes, pumpkin seeds and a pinch of sea salt, to taste.

Savoury Buckwheat Pancakes with Sun-dried Tomatoes and Parma Ham

A savoury breakfast that doesn't scrimp on flavour! Enjoy these as a lazy weekend brunch to really impress!

50g buckwheat flour

1 large free-range egg

150ml water

coconut oil, for frying

4 slices of Parma ham

1 small handful of fresh spinach

6 sun-dried tomatoes, drained and cut into small pieces

sea salt and freshly ground black pepper

SERVES 4

1. Sift the flour into a large bowl, create a well in the centre then break in the egg. Using a whisk, gradually add the water and continue to whisk until the mixture has completely combined and has the consistency of thin cream.

2. Add a pinch of salt and pepper and stir through.

3. Heat a small amount of coconut oil in a frying pan and pour in a quarter of the mixture to fry.

4. Once the base of the pancake has set, add a slice of Parma ham, a small amount of spinach and tomatoes to one half, and fold the pancake over.

5. Leave to cook for another 30 seconds before plating up and repeating with the remaining mixture.

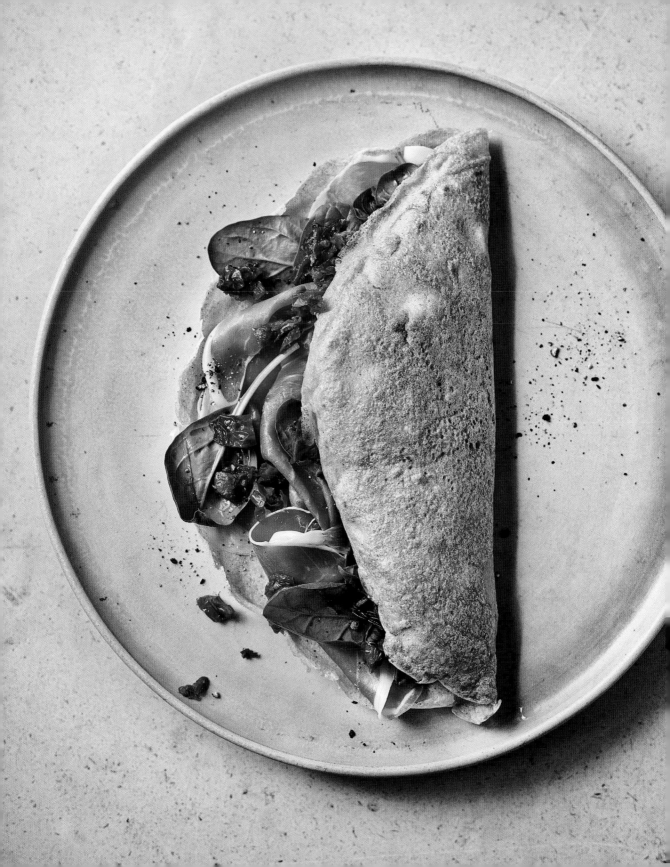

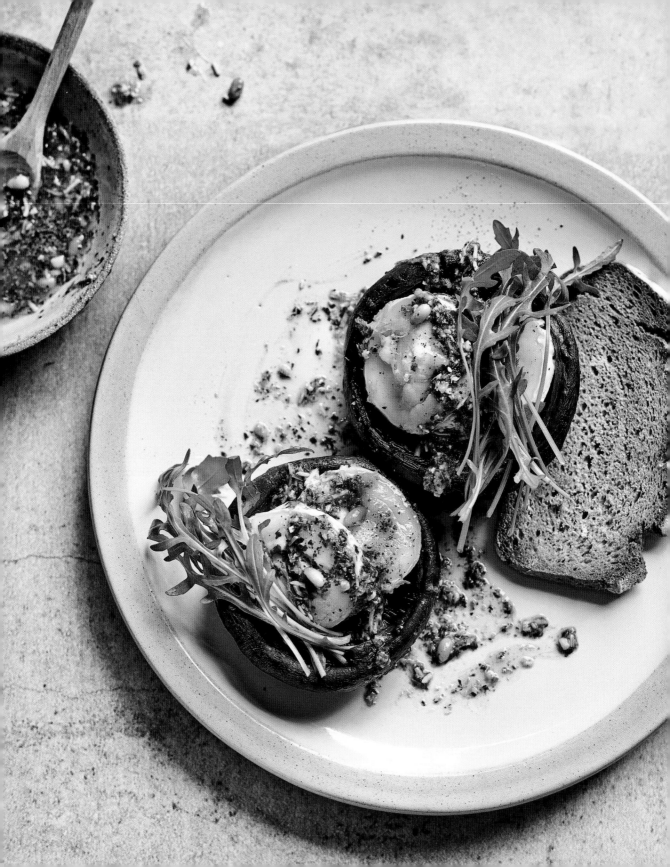

Grilled Portobello Mushrooms with Goat's Cheese, Pesto and Rocket

Eggs aren't for everyone, so this is excellent as a delicious alternative. You just can't beat gooey goat's cheese paired with the peppery rocket.

1 tsp coconut oil

4 large portobello mushrooms

200g goat's cheese, cut into
   1-2cm slices

grated zest of ¼ lemon

50g rocket

2 tbsp pesto

toasted rye bread (optional)

sea salt and freshly ground
   black pepper

SERVES 2

1. Preheat the grill.
2. Melt the coconut oil until it is a liquid then coat the mushrooms in the oil and season. Place them onto a foil-lined tray and cook under the grill for about 10 minutes or until softened.
3. Slice your goat's cheese into 1-2cm slices, top with a pinch of lemon zest then place on the cooked mushrooms. Put them back under the grill for a few minutes.
4. Remove the mushrooms and plate them up, topping them with a handful of rocket and a good drizzle of pesto.
5. Serve with some toasted rye bread, if using.

Smoked Mackerel Pâté on Toasted Pumpernickel

Make this pâté in bulk to not only ensure you have a breakfast rich in omega-3 and omega-6 fatty acids, but also as a great snack to curb those cravings!

1 smoked mackerel fillet, broken into pieces

1 tsp grated lemon zest

2 tbsp quark

1 tsp chopped fresh chives

50g rocket (optional)

2 slices of toasted pumpernickel or similar bread (sourdough, rye)

sea salt and freshly ground black pepper

SERVES 1

1. In a food processor or blender, blitz the smoked mackerel, lemon zest and quark with a good pinch of salt and pepper, until smooth.

2. Stir in the chives.

3. Spread the pumpernickel slices with the pâté and top with a good helping of rocket, if using.

Raspberry and Pomegranate Pancake with Coconut 'Cream'

I absolutely love coconut, and this sweet breakfast hit is the most delicious combination of tangy fruit with smooth coconut cream.

½ banana, mashed

2 free-range eggs

½ tsp ground cinnamon

coconut oil, for frying

100g raspberries

50g pomegranate seeds

½ tsp coconut flavouring

50g desiccated coconut

150g quark or Greek yogurt

SERVES 1

1. Mix together the banana, eggs and cinnamon until fully combined.

2. In a non-stick frying pan, heat a small amount of coconut oil and then pour in the pancake mixture.

3. Once the base has slightly set, add the fresh raspberries and pomegranate seeds to one side of the pancake then fold the pancake over. Leave to cook for a further few minutes.

4. To make the coconut cream, add the coconut flavouring and desiccated coconut to the quark, or yogurt, and stir until completely combined.

5. Plate up the pancake, top with coconut cream and serve.

LUNCH

When you're midway through a busy day, it's always nice to know that there is something delicious waiting for you to eat to keep energy levels up and hunger at bay. Most, if not all, of you have busy lives, and lunch can sometimes be an awkward one. Prepping food in advance will ensure that you don't find yourself at a loss and running to the nearest supermarket for a makeshift lunch.

Sacrificing an hour of your Sunday to prepare some delicious lunches and snacks for the week will be totally worth it, despite it perhaps feeling like a slight chore at first. As the saying goes, 'Failing to prepare is preparing to fail,' and this certainly holds true in my opinion. Planning and preparing all you need to stay focused and on the plan will mean temptation won't rear its head – you will eat well and feel full, as well as avoiding that dangerous afternoon-biscuit slump.

Chilli Beef Lettuce Wraps

A great low-carb lunch – perfect for rest days!

1 tsp coconut oil, for frying

1 red chilli, deseeded and finely diced

½ red onion, finely diced

400g beef mince

3 tbsp tamari

1 garlic clove, crushed

1 handful of fresh parsley, finely chopped

1 lime

1 baby gem lettuce, leaves separated

sea salt and freshly ground black pepper

SERVES 2

1. Place a pan over a medium heat with the coconut oil.
2. Add the chilli and red onion and cook gently for a few minutes before adding the beef. Season with salt and pepper.
3. Once the beef is completely browned, break it up with a wooden spoon, combine the tamari and garlic and stir through the beef so that it is all coated.
4. Place the beef in a bowl and scatter over the parsley and a dash of fresh lime juice.
5. Serve in lettuce wraps and enjoy.

Harissa Chicken with Pomegranate, Cauliflower Rice and Coriander

Cauliflower rice is perfect for rest days when you need fewer carbs. This lunch is great for making in bulk, so you can have some leftovers for lunch too.

2 skinless chicken breasts

2 tsp harissa paste

coconut oil, for frying

1 large head of cauliflower

1 small handful of fresh
   coriander, chopped

100g pomegranate seeds

small pinch of garlic salt

1 tbsp flaked almonds

SERVES 2

1. Place the chicken breasts, harissa paste and a small amount of coconut oil in a large sandwich bag and gently rub until both breasts are coated.

2. Heat a small amount of coconut oil in a large frying pan then add the coated chicken breasts to the pan and cook over a medium heat.

3. Meanwhile, remove the core and stalks from the cauliflower and pulse the florets in a food processor to make grains the size of rice.

4. Place the cauliflower rice in a heatproof dish and cover with clingfilm, ensuring you pierce a few holes in the film, and microwave for about 7 minutes on high.

5. Once cooked, remove the clingfilm, stir in the coriander, pomegranate seeds and garlic salt and plate up before topping with the cooked chicken breast and a small sprinkling of flaked almonds.

Chilli Prawn Salad with Red Cabbage and Carrot Slaw

A simple, delicious and crunchy lunch with prawns added for a maximum protein punch.

FOR THE SALAD

175g red cabbage, shredded

175g carrots, shredded

1 small handful of fresh coriander, chopped

1 small handful of fresh mint, chopped

4 tbsp unsalted peanuts

200g cooked large peeled prawns

FOR THE DRESSING

1 red chilli, deseeded and finely chopped

1 garlic clove, crushed

3 tbsp lime juice

SERVES 2

1. Begin by combining the red cabbage, carrot, mint and coriander in a serving bowl.

2. In a dry pan, fry the peanuts until lightly browned and toasted then leave to cool. Break into smaller chunks using a knife or place into a small sandwich bag and crush with a rolling pin.

3. Top the salad with the prawns and peanuts.

4. Mix the dressing ingredients together and drizzle over the salad before giving it a good mix to ensure all the ingredients are coated.

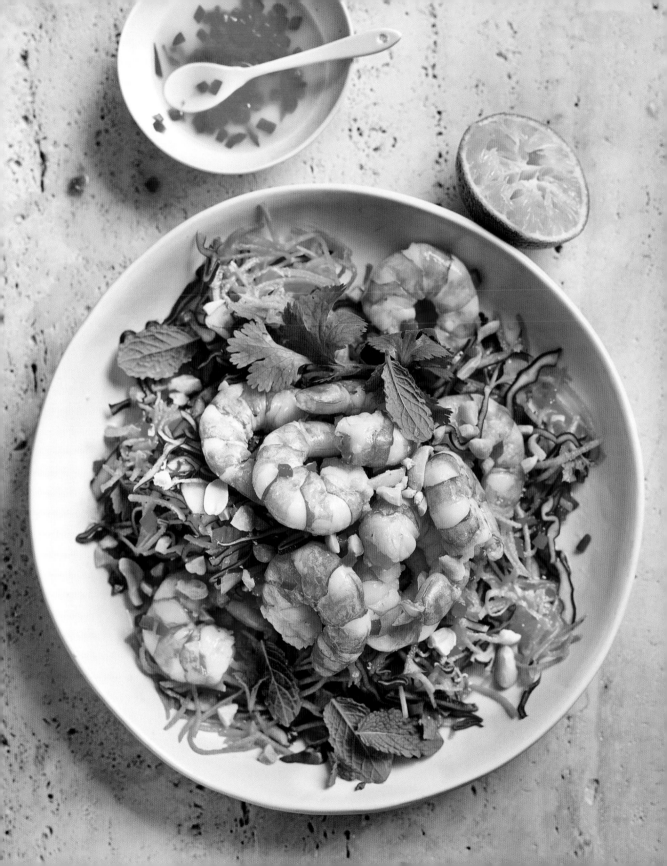

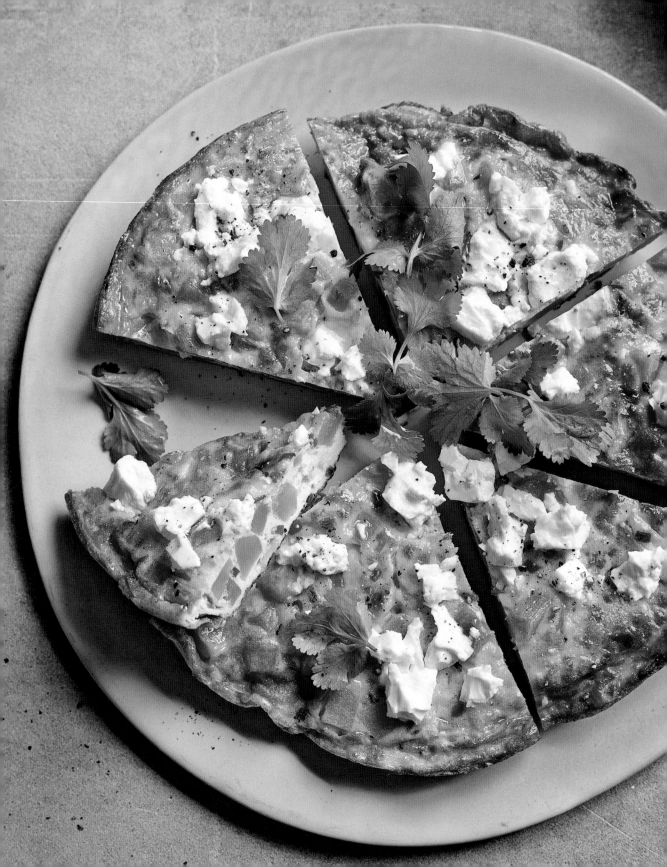

Butternut Squash, Chilli and Feta Frittata

The perfect meal to last all week, pack a few slices for lunch on the go.

1 tsp coconut oil, for frying

1 small red onion, finely diced

400g butternut squash, cut into small cubes

2 red chillies, deseeded and finely chopped

1 garlic clove, crushed

2 tbsp cider vinegar

6 free-range eggs

150g feta cheese, in crumbled chunks

1 small handful of coriander, to serve

SERVES 2

1. Preheat the grill.
2. Heat the coconut oil in a large frying pan then add the red onion and butternut squash and cook for about 15 minutes over a medium heat until soft.
3. Mix the chilli, garlic and cider vinegar in a bowl then add to the frying pan with the squash. Stir until it is all lightly covered.
4. Pour the eggs over the mixture and scatter over the feta cheese in even chunks across the pan. Cook until the base is set, then place under the grill until the top is completely cooked.
5. Sprinkle with the coriander before serving.

Blackened Cod with Radish and Red Cabbage Slaw

This is brilliant if you want something light and easy to digest. I particularly love it in the summer.

8-10 radishes, thinly
    sliced

100g red cabbage, shredded

1 red onion, thinly sliced

1 small handful of fresh
    coriander

juice of 1 lime

1 tsp smoked paprika

1 tsp ground cumin

½ tsp garlic salt

200g cod fillet

½ tsp coconut oil, for
    frying

SERVES 1

1. In a large bowl, mix together the radish, red cabbage, red onion and two-thirds of the coriander and stir through the lime juice.

2. Mix the spices and salt together and coat the fish until completely covered.

3. Heat the coconut oil in a frying pan until very hot then fry the cod over a high heat for about 2 minutes on each side before serving alongside the slaw with the remaining coriander.

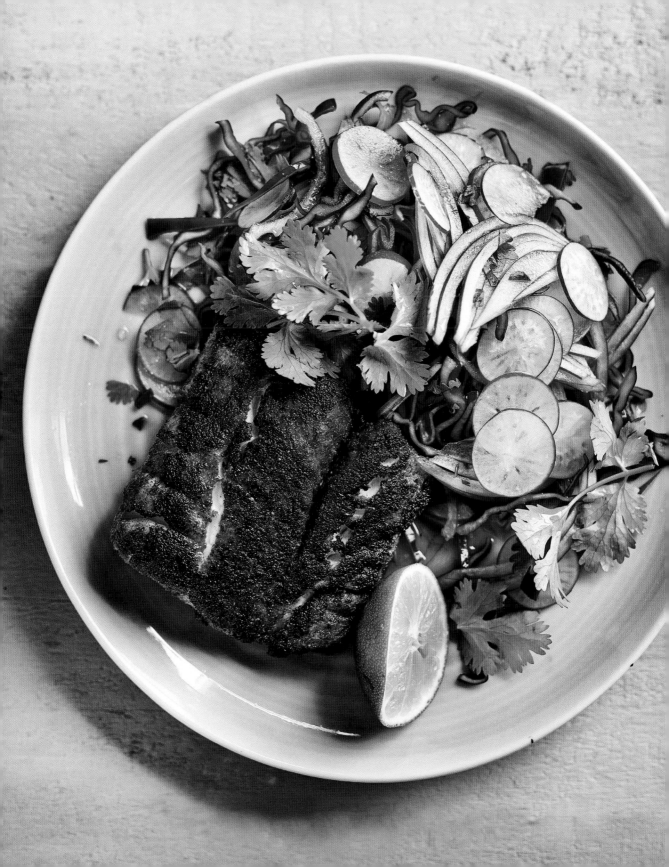

Prawn, Watermelon and Feta Salad

Another great one to make in bulk and keep in the fridge. It is brilliant for lunch the next day.

200g raw large peeled prawns

coconut oil, for frying

100g Tenderstem broccoli

200g watermelon, cut into chunks

1 small handful of fresh mint

200g feta cheese, crumbled into chunks

FOR THE DRESSING

1 tbsp extra virgin olive oil

juice of 1 lemon

sea salt and freshly ground black pepper

SERVES 2

1. Mix the dressing ingredients with a little salt and pepper, then pour 1 tablespoon over the prawns and leave to marinate for about 15 minutes.

2. Meanwhile, heat a small amount of coconut oil in a pan and gently fry the broccoli for 3 to 4 minutes, then leave to cool.

3. Once cooled, arrange in a bowl with the watermelon, mint leaves and crumbled feta.

4. Heat a small amount of coconut oil in a frying pan until very hot then fry your marinated prawns until fully pink and cooked. Add to the rest of the salad.

5. Drizzle over the remaining dressing and gently toss together until everything is covered.

Toasted Rye Bread with Pea Purée and Mackerel

A light bite that makes a great lunch-on-the-go.

200g frozen peas

½ tsp dried mint

1 tbsp Greek yogurt

1 slice of rye bread

125g tin mackerel fillets in brine, drained, or smoked mackerel

chilli flakes (optional)

sea salt and freshly ground black pepper

SERVES 1

1. Place the peas and dried mint and a little salt and pepper in a saucepan and cover with cold water. Simmer for about 5 minutes or until slightly soft, then drain.

2. Place the peas and Greek yogurt in a food processor and blitz into a rough purée.

3. Toast the rye bread, spread the purée onto the bread, then top with the mackerel fillets.

4. Finish with a pinch of chilli flakes, if desired, and a good grind of salt and pepper.

Teriyaki Steak Skewers with Asian-style Greens

I love the Asian flavours in this dish and the steak is a great source of protein for post-workout fuel.

FOR THE MARINADE

1 tbsp soy sauce

1 tbsp mirin

1 tbsp honey

1 thumb-sized piece of
    fresh ginger, grated

400g lean diced steak, with
    fat trimmed

1 large pak choi, shredded

1 large handful of kale,
    shredded

1 spring onion, sliced

½ cucumber, deseeded and
    diced

1 tbsp sherry vinegar

1 tsp olive oil

1 tsp soy sauce

1 red chilli, deseeded and
    thinly sliced (optional)

SERVES 2

1. Create your marinade by mixing the soy, mirin and honey with half of the ginger and pour it over the steak, leaving to marinate for about an hour.

2. Mix the pak choi, kale, spring onion and cucumber and toss with the sherry vinegar, the olive oil, the remaining ginger and the soy sauce and assemble in a serving bowl.

3. Using small skewers, thread about four steak pieces on to each skewer and then sear in a hot frying pan for about 2 minutes on each side.

4. Once all the steak has been cooked, serve with the salad. Finish with a sprinkling of chilli, if using.

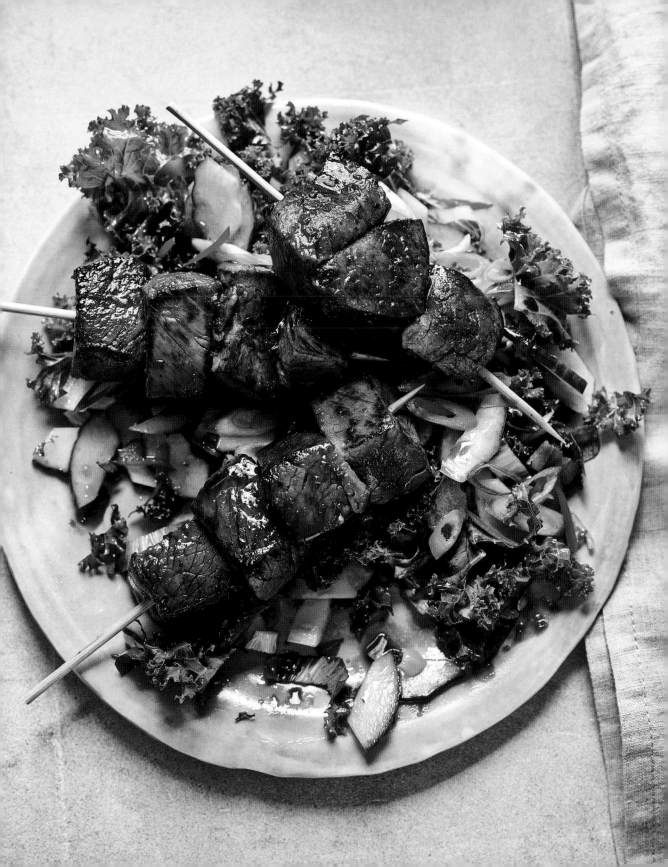

Smile, Sparkle, Shine

Super-simple Prawn Curry with Rice

Because, who doesn't love a curry? Another great alternative to those calorie-laden takeaways.

coconut oil, for frying

1 garlic clove, crushed

1 small chunk of fresh
  ginger, grated

2 tbsp curry paste

400ml reduced-fat coconut
  milk

200g raw large peeled
  prawns

1 bag of microwaveable rice

1 small handful of fresh
  coriander

SERVES 2

1. Heat a little coconut oil in a pan, cook the garlic and ginger for a couple of minutes then stir in the curry paste and cook for a minute.

2. Add the coconut milk to the pan and bring to a simmer.

3. Add the prawns to the pan and cook until pink and cooked through.

4. While the prawns are cooking, heat your rice in the microwave following the packet instructions.

5. Plate up the rice and top with a portion of the prawn curry and some fresh coriander.

Simple Salmon Fishcakes with Carrot Chips and Smashed Avocado

These are a wonderful alternative to frozen, supermarket-bought fishcakes and are great cold the next day too. This is a real treat lunch plate for me.

2 carrots, cut into batons

coconut oil, for greasing and frying

2 salmon fillets

1 free-range egg, beaten

½ red onion, finely diced

1 tsp smoked paprika

pinch of chilli flakes

4 tbsp buckwheat flour

1 ripe avocado, halved, stone removed and flesh mashed

1 tsp lemon juice

sea salt and freshly ground black pepper

SERVES 2

1. Preheat the oven to 180°C/350°F/Gas Mark 4.

2. Using your hands, massage the carrot batons with a little coconut oil before placing them on a foil-lined tray and seasoning with salt and pepper. Place in the oven and cook for about 20 minutes, or until slightly golden.

3. Cook the salmon fillets, either by pan-frying them in a little coconut oil or in the oven.

4. Once cooked, leave to cool slightly then, in a mixing bowl, mash the salmon with the egg, onion, paprika, chilli flakes and half of the buckwheat flour until all the ingredients are completely combined.

5. Using your hands, form round patties from the mixture and then coat in the remaining buckwheat flour and leave to stand on a plate.

6. Heat a small amount of coconut oil in a non-stick frying pan and place the patties into the pan to fry. Once one side is slightly browned, flip them using a spatula and cook on the other side.

7. Serve the patties alongside some smashed avocado drizzled with a little lemon juice, and the roasted carrot chips.

Crispy Harissa Salmon with Cucumber and Mint Raita and New Potatoes

Light, delicious and refreshing, this is the ultimate taste bud adventure..

2 tbsp Greek yogurt

½ cucumber, finely chopped

1 large handful of fresh
   mint, chopped

½ green chilli, deseeded and
   finely chopped

1 tsp harissa paste

1 tsp agave nectar

2 salmon fillets

coconut oil, for frying

8-10 new potatoes, steamed
   and sliced

100g Tenderstem broccoli,
   steamed

juice of ¼ lemon

sea salt and freshly ground
   black pepper

SERVES 2

1. Mix together the yogurt, cucumber, mint, chilli and a good pinch of salt and pepper until fully combined.

2. Mix the harissa paste with the agave nectar until well combined and coat the salmon fillets with the mixture.

3. Heat a small amount of coconut oil in a non-stick frying pan and add the salmon fillets, skin side down. Leave to fry for 2 to 3 minutes before turning them over and leaving to fry for a further 1 to 2 minutes.

4. Once the salmon is cooked, assemble the sliced new potatoes with the broccoli. Top with the salmon and a generous helping of raita before finishing with a squeeze of fresh lemon juice.

Jerk Chicken with Mango Salsa

A super-easy dish that is perfect for those lunches when you are short on time. It is super-nutritious and delicious. This recipe makes a generous portion of salsa - ideal for adding to leftovers the following day.

2 skinless chicken breasts

2 tbsp jerk paste

$\frac{1}{2}$ mango, peeled, stone removed and diced into small chunks

$\frac{1}{2}$ red onion, finely diced

1 large salad tomato, deseeded and finely diced

$\frac{1}{4}$ cucumber, deseeded and finely diced

$\frac{1}{2}$ red chilli, deseeded and finely diced

drizzle of lime juice

1 small handful of fresh mint, chopped

1 small handful of fresh coriander, chopped

cooked rice, to serve (optional)

sea salt and freshly ground black pepper

SERVES 2

1. Preheat the grill.

2. Brush the chicken breasts with the jerk paste and season well before placing onto a foil-lined tray and under the grill for about 20 minutes or until fully cooked.

3. Meanwhile, mix the mango, red onion, tomato, cucumber and chilli, drizzle with a little lime juice and season, then stir through the mint and coriander.

4. Once the chicken is cooked, slice and serve with a heaped tablespoon of mango salsa and rice, if using.

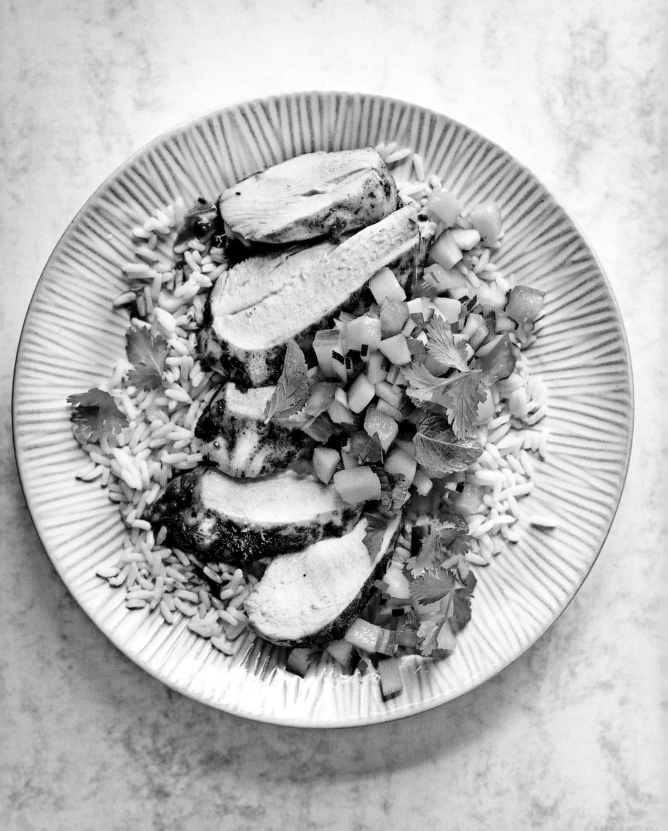

Roasted Tomatoes and Avocado on Sourdough Toast

Whether you're trying out a meat-free Monday or you just feel like some pure veggie goodness, this won't disappoint!

8-10 cherry tomatoes, halved

½ tsp melted coconut oil

1 ripe avocado, halved, stone removed and peeled

juice of ½ lemon

2 slices of thick sourdough bread, toasted

balsamic glaze, for drizzling

50g rocket

sea salt and freshly ground black pepper

SERVES 1-2

1. Preheat the grill.

2. Place the tomatoes on a foil-lined tray and drizzle with the coconut oil. Season well and place under the grill to cook for about 10 minutes.

3. Using a fork, mash the avocado and mix with the lemon juice and a pinch of salt and pepper. Spread evenly onto your toasted sourdough.

4. Once the tomatoes are cooked, place them on top of the toast and avocado, drizzle with a little balsamic glaze and serve topped with rocket.

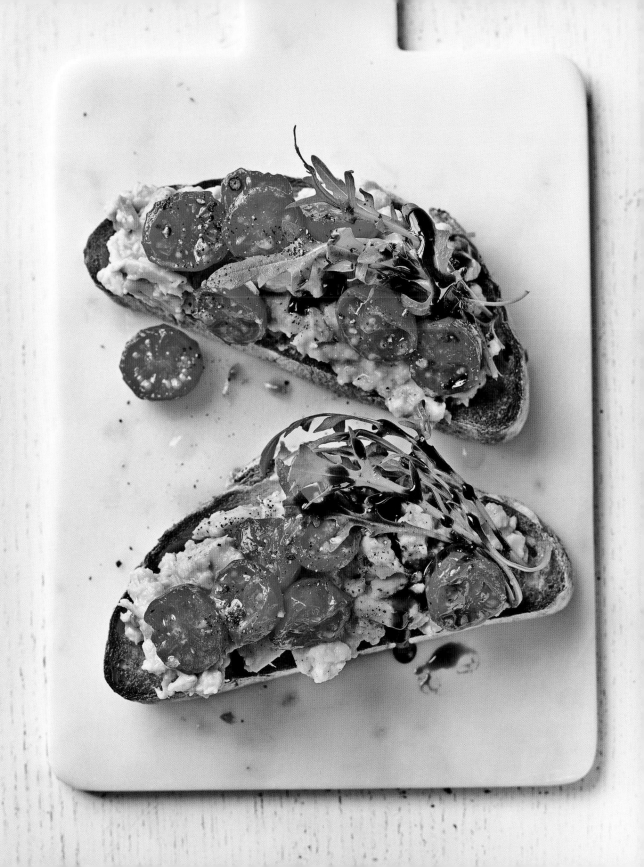

DINNER

My favourite meal of the day. I always like to have a plentiful dinner, something that is going to refuel me after being on the go all day and will ensure I sleep well.

I usually reserve a large portion of my daily calorie allowance for my dinner, and build each evening meal around a source of good-quality protein such as fish or meat. My recipes are all completely flexible, giving you the freedom to add in or remove ingredients where necessary. If you find yourself extra hungry on a particular day, or have had an intense workout, try adding in some extra delicious sweet potato fries. If you are on a rest day, you can swap regular rice for cauliflower rice, which works perfectly as a low-carb alternative. My saying when it comes to cooking is 'There is never a problem, only a solution,' so don't be afraid to experiment with extra flavours and ingredients. Making these meals personal to you will mean you're far more likely to sustain this new way of eating and keep cravings at bay.

Warm Lentil, Roasted Veg and Feta Salad with Grilled Lamb Steaks

Lentils are high in fibre and are a great source of both protein and carbohydrate. I love this salad, which can be enjoyed all year round for a plentiful evening meal.

2 medium courgettes, peeled and cut into chunks

150g butternut squash, peeled and cut into chunks

2 medium carrots, peeled and cut into chunks

10 cherry tomatoes, halved

1 tsp coconut oil, melted

2 lamb leg steaks

250g cooked lentils

100g feta cheese, crumbled

needles from 1 sprig fresh rosemary, chopped

juice of ½ lemon

sea salt and freshly ground black pepper

SERVES 2

1. Preheat the oven to 180°C/350°F/Gas Mark 4.

2. Lay the vegetables in a roasting dish and drizzle with the coconut oil. Season well, then place in the oven to roast for about 30 minutes, until slightly browned and tender. Remove from the oven and set aside to cool.

3. Preheat the grill. Lay the lamb steaks on a foil-lined tray and season well on both sides, before placing under the grill to cook for about 3 minutes on each side.

4. Heat the lentils in the microwave then divide them equally between two plates.

5. Top with a generous helping of roasted vegetables, then add the grilled lamb steaks.

6. Sprinkle over the crumbled feta, rosemary and finish with a drizzle of lemon juice.

Caramelized Lemon and Herb Salmon with Sweet Potato and Feta

Salmon is not only a tasty source of protein, it is also full of essential fatty acids and is a real staple in my diet. This dish, with its sweet potato and feta, provides a combination of protein, carbohydrates and fats to refuel post workout or replenish you after a busy day.

2 salmon fillets

coconut oil, for greasing and frying

2 lemons, 1 cut into thick slices, and 1 juiced

2 garlic cloves

450g sweet potatoes, peeled and cut into 5mm-thick rounds

20g fresh parsley, finely chopped

200ml extra virgin olive oil

½ red onion, finely chopped

40g feta cheese

sea salt and freshly ground black pepper

SERVES 2

1. Preheat the oven to 190°C/375°F/Gas Mark 5.
2. Score the skin of the salmon fillets with a sharp knife, rub with a little coconut oil and season with salt and a good few grinds of pepper. Place on 2 large sheets of foil.
3. Heat a 20p-sized piece of coconut oil in a frying pan, then place the lemon slices in the pan. Fry until golden, then remove the pan from the heat and set aside for 2 to 3 minutes.
4. Place the caramelized lemon slices on the salmon fillets, throw in the garlic cloves then wrap the foil around the salmon, sealing the edges together to create a parcel. Place the parcels on a baking tray then put in the middle of the oven to cook for 15 to 20 minutes. Remove the salmon parcel from the oven and leave it to stand for about 10 minutes.
5. While the salmon is baking in the oven, put the sliced sweet potatoes in a pan, cover with boiling water and simmer over a medium heat for about 10 minutes or until soft.
6. Combine the parsley with the olive oil, lemon juice and onion and season with a little salt and pepper.
7. When the sweet potato is cooked, drain then assemble the slices in a dish. Drizzle with the parsley and olive oil dressing. Place the cooked salmon fillets on top, crumble over the feta and serve.

Warm Roasted Butternut Squash, Kale and Feta Salad with Pomegranate

A quick, easy and nutritious dinner with the delicious combination of tangy feta and sweet pomegranate.

FOR THE SALAD

150g butternut squash, peeled and cut into small chunks

coconut oil

1 small red onion, finely diced

1 large handful of kale, tough stems removed and leaves torn

7-10 small tomatoes, halved

40g feta cheese, crumbled

50g pomegranate seeds

sea salt

FOR THE DRESSING

3 tbsp extra virgin olive oil

1 tbsp cider vinegar

1 garlic clove, finely crushed

sea salt and freshly ground black pepper

SERVES 1

1. Preheat the oven to 180°C/350°F/Gas Mark 4.

2. Using your hands, take a piece of coconut oil (the size of a 20p coin) and massage the butternut squash until it is all lightly covered. Sprinkle with a pinch of salt then place on a foil-lined tray. Roast for 20 to 30 minutes, tossing half way through the cooking time.

3. Heat a small amount of coconut oil in a frying pan, add the red onion, kale and tomatoes and cook gently for about 5 minutes.

4. Once cooked, assemble the kale, red onion and tomatoes in a dish and add the cooked butternut squash, crumbled feta and pomegranate seeds.

5. To make the dressing, mix the olive oil, cider vinegar and garlic together. Add a pinch of salt and pepper and mix again before pouring over the salad.

Optional extras

1. Need more protein? Add chicken. Cube a chicken breast and cook in a frying pan with a little coconut oil, a squeeze of lemon and some garlic salt.

2. Need more carbohydrates? Swap the butternut squash for sweet potato or cooked lentils.

3. Need more fats? Try adding some fresh avocado.

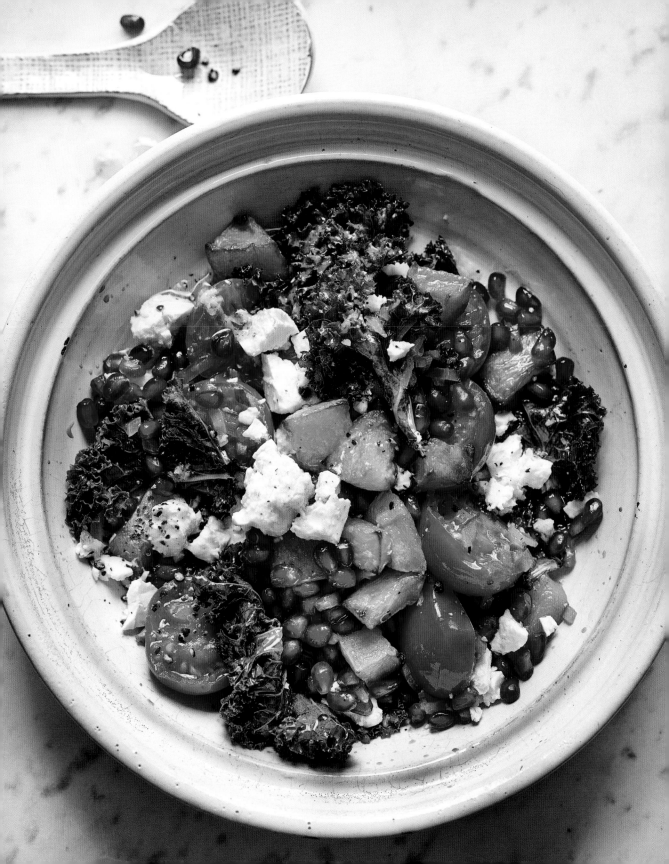

Grilled Cajun Salmon with Rice and Tenderstem Broccoli

Super simple, with a little spice, this recipe can be made in bulk and enjoyed for lunch the next day too!

2 salmon fillets

1 tsp paprika

½ tsp cayenne pepper

½ tsp garlic powder

¼ tsp ground cumin

200g basmati rice (or similar)

100g Tenderstem broccoli

squeeze of lemon juice (optional)

SERVES 2

1. Preheat the grill.

2. Begin by mixing all the spices together.

3. Place the salmon fillets on a foil-lined tray and sprinkle some of the spice mix over the salmon until completely covered.

4. Place the salmon under the grill to cook for about 12 minutes.

5. Meanwhile, bring a pan of water to the boil then add the broccoli to cook for a few minutes, until tender. Drain and place on two plates.

6. Cook the rice according to the packet instructions. Once cooked, mix any leftover spices through the rice for added flavour. Add the rice to the plates, place the cooked salmon on top and serve with a squeeze of fresh lemon juice, if you like.

Sea Bass with Roasted Vegetables

Teamed with roasted vegetables, this fish is low in calories so it makes a great light dinner for rest days.

coconut oil, for greasing
    and frying
1 red pepper, deseeded and
    sliced
1 small red onion, sliced
1 tsp chopped fresh thyme
1 tsp garlic paste
2 sea bass fillets
juice of ¼ lemon
sea salt and freshly ground
    black pepper

SERVES 2

1. Preheat the oven to 200°C/400°F/Gas Mark 6 and line a roasting dish with foil.

2. Using your hands, take a small amount of coconut oil and rub the vegetables so they all have a light coating, then place in the roasting dish and sprinkle with the chopped thyme and a little salt and pepper.

3. Place in the oven to cook for 25 to 30 minutes.

4. When the vegetables are almost cooked, heat a small amount of coconut oil and the garlic paste in a frying pan until very hot.

5. Season the sea bass fillets and then place them, skin side down, into the hot pan to fry. Cook until the skin is crispy and golden and then flip and cook for a further minute.

6. Plate up the cooked sea bass and roasted vegetables and drizzle with lemon juice.

Grilled Halloumi, Rocket and Courgette Salad

I love halloumi. This salad is great for a warm summer evening, and is wonderful for sharing.

FOR THE SALAD

1 tbsp pine nuts

100g rocket

100g fresh peas

8-10 cherry tomatoes, halved

2 large courgettes

100g halloumi

FOR THE DRESSING

juice of 1 lemon

3 tbsp extra virgin olive oil

pinch of sea salt and freshly ground black pepper

SERVES 2

1. Toast the pine nuts in a dry pan over a high heat until slightly browned and then tip into a bowl.

2. Next, assemble the rocket in a serving bowl and toss over the fresh peas, tomatoes and toasted pine nuts.

3. Using a peeler or spiralizer, slice the courgettes into thin ribbons and assemble on top of the rocket.

4. Cut the halloumi into thin slices and fry for a few minutes on each side in the frying pan until golden and crispy.

5. Combine the dressing ingredients and drizzle over the salad, tossing it gently until everything is covered.

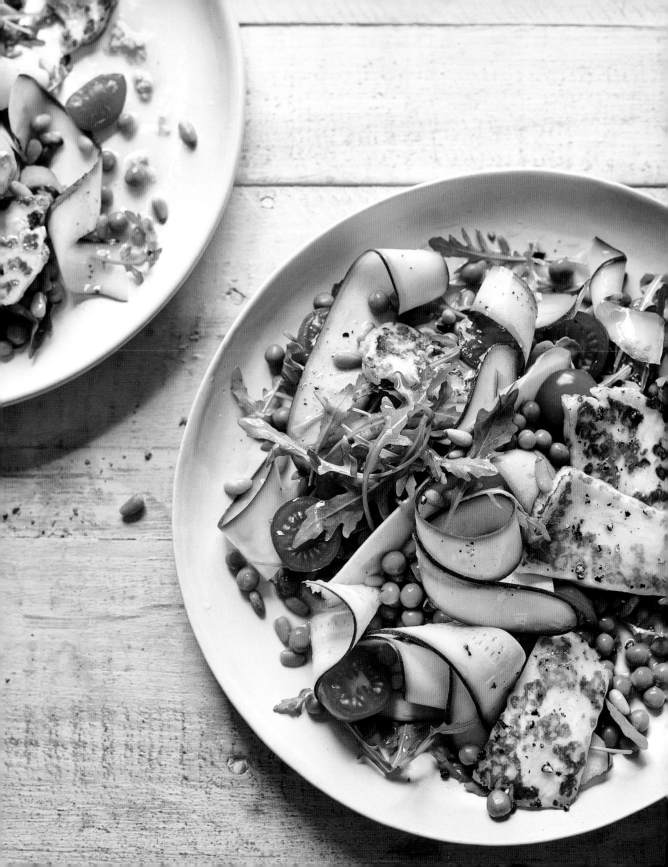

Spicy Chilli Con Carne with Smashed Avocado and Asparagus

I love the spice in this warming dish. Paired with the creamy avocado, this makes for one of my all-time favourite dinners. It can also be made in bulk and is equally nice as leftovers.

½ tsp coconut oil

2 garlic cloves, crushed

1 large onion, finely chopped

400g minced beef

1 red pepper, cut into small
    chunks

2 tsp ground cumin

1 tsp ground coriander

½ tsp dried oregano

1 tbsp tomato purée

400g tinned chopped tomatoes

400g tinedn kidney beans,
    drained

100g asparagus spears

1 large ripe avocado, halved
and stone removed

juice of ¼ lemon

sea salt and black pepper

1 small handful of fresh
    coriander, to serve

SERVES 2

1. Heat a small amount of coconut oil in a pan and fry the onion and garlic until softened, then add your mince and fry off until brown. Add the spices and cook for a few minutes, stirring occasionally.

2. Add the tomato purée, chopped tomatoes, peppers and kidney beans and leave to simmer gently for about 30 minutes.

3. When the beef is almost ready, in a separate frying pan, heat a small amount of coconut oil and fry off the asparagus with a generous helping of black pepper until soft.

4. Mash the avocado using a fork and mix through the lemon juice, a pinch of salt and a generous helping of pepper.

5. Serve the mince topped with a large spoonful of smashed avocado, a little fresh coriander and the asparagus.

Mozzarella and Rocket Cauliflower-crust Pizza

A great twist on something that used to be a real staple in my diet. This pizza is great for entertaining and enjoying with friends for an impressive and healthy dinner!

½ large cauliflower, broken into florets

1 free-range egg, beaten

50g Parmesan cheese

½ garlic clove, crushed

coconut oil, for frying

250g tomato passata

1 small handful of fresh basil

50-60g light mozzarella, sliced

1 small handful of rocket

chilli flakes (optional)

sea salt

SERVES 2

1. Preheat the oven to 200°C/400°F/Gas Mark 6.

2. Cook the cauliflower in a saucepan of boiling water for about 4 minutes before draining and removing any excess water. Place in a food processor and whizz until it resembles small rice-like pieces.

3. Place the cauliflower, egg and Parmesan cheese in a large mixing bowl and mix until combined.

4. Spread the mixture onto a foil-lined, lightly oiled baking sheet and press until it resembles a pizza base.

5. Bake in the oven for 15 to 20 minutes or until it is golden and feels firm.

6. While the pizza base is cooking, fry the garlic in a little coconut oil before adding the passata. Leave this to simmer gently, then add the basil and reduce the heat until it has thickened and can be spread onto the pizza base.

7. Once the base has cooked, spread the tomato sauce onto the base, then add the mozzarella slices and place back in the oven for a further 10 minutes.

8. Remove from the oven and top with fresh rocket, a pinch of sea salt, and chilli flakes, if using.

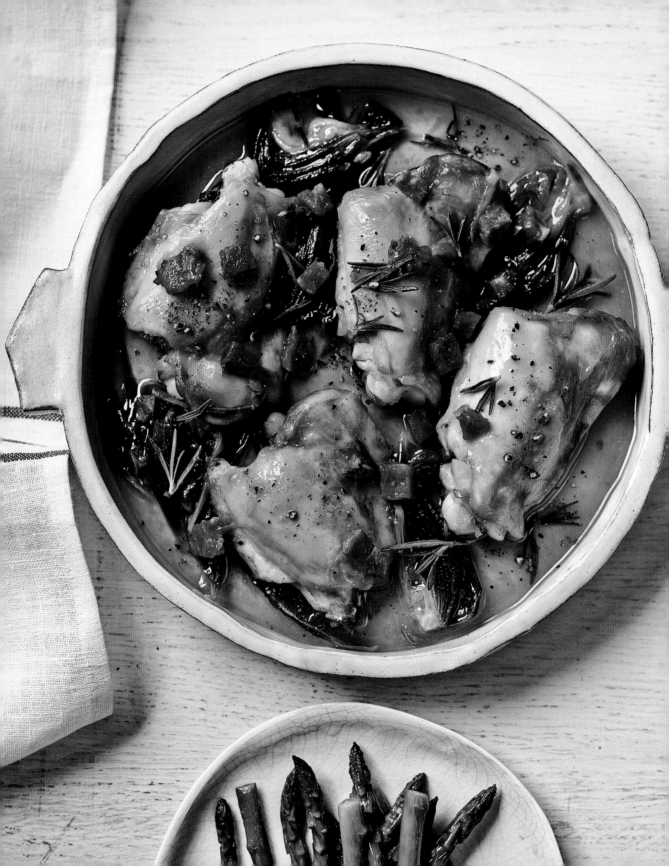

One-pot Chicken and Chorizo

One for all the family, this is a versatile recipe that can be prepped in advance and any leftovers stored for lunches. The chorizo provides a delicious amount of flavour to really spice up this chicken dish.

coconut oil, for greasing and frying

4 skinless chicken thighs

1 small red onion, cut into wedges

100ml chicken stock

30g chorizo, cut into small chunks

1 tsp chopped fresh rosemary

100g asparagus

sea salt and freshly ground black pepper

SERVES 2

1. Preheat the oven to 200°C/400°F/Gas Mark 6.
2. Lightly grease a baking dish with a little coconut oil and then place the chicken thighs into the dish.
3. Tuck the onion wedges underneath the thighs, then season each thigh well with a good grind of pepper and a pinch of salt.
4. Pour the chicken stock into the dish then place in the oven to cook for about 30 minutes.
5. Once 30 minutes is up, add the chorizo then place back in the oven and cook for a further 15 minutes.
6. Remove the chicken from the oven and top with the rosemary. Reduce the heat slightly, give the dish a good stir, before placing back into the oven for a further 10 minutes.
7. Meanwhile, heat a small amount of coconut oil in a frying pan and gently fry the asparagus, seasoning it with salt and pepper. Cook until slightly browned and softened then remove and serve alongside the chicken.

Roasted Vegetable and Couscous Salad with Chilli and Lime Chicken

FOR THE MARINADE

2 garlic cloves, crushed

¼ tsp chilli paste

¼ tsp cayenne pepper

1 tsp paprika

zest and juice of 1 lime

1 tbsp coconut oil, melted

2 large skinless chicken
    breasts

FOR THE ROASTED VEGETABLES

1 red onion, diced

1 courgette, cut into chunks

1 red pepper, deseeded and
    diced

1 small sweet potato, diced

coconut oil, melted, for
    drizzling

200g couscous

400ml boiling water

25g butter

grated zest and juice of ½
    lemon

1 small handful of fresh
    basil, chopped

sea salt and freshly ground
    black pepper

SERVES 2

I always love trying new ways of enjoying chicken and this dish definitely provides flavour in abundance, while also being a great post-workout refuel.

1. Begin by making the marinade. Combine all the ingredients in a bowl then, using your hands, coat each chicken breast until completely covered. Place on a foil-lined baking tray.

2. Preheat the oven to 200°C/400°F/Gas Mark 6.

3. On a separate foil-lined baking tray, spread the vegetables out, drizzle them with a little coconut oil and season with a pinch of salt and pepper. Place the chicken and vegetables into the oven to cook for about 30 minutes.

4. Once the chicken is cooked through and the vegetables are starting to brown slightly around the edges, remove from the oven and leave to stand.

5. Meanwhile, put the couscous in a heatproof bowl and pour over the boiling water and add the butter, lemon juice and zest. Stir well. Cover the dish and leave it to stand for 5 to 6 minutes, or until all the liquid is absorbed.

6. Add the roasted vegetables and chopped basil and give everything a good stir. Top with the chicken and serve.

Warming Winter Shepherd's Pie

Comfort food at its finest. This is a great remake of the old family favourite and a real winter warmer.

coconut oil, for frying

400g extra-lean beef mince

1 red onion, finely diced

2 carrots, finely chopped

2 celery sticks, finely chopped

2 garlic cloves, crushed

¼ tsp ground cinnamon

1 small handful of fresh rosemary, chopped

200g tinned chopped tomatoes

2 sweet potatoes, chopped into cubes

2 tbsp Greek yogurt

sea salt and freshly ground black pepper

Serves 4

1. Preheat the oven to 200°C/400°F/Gas Mark 6.

2. Heat a small amount of coconut oil in a large frying pan, and brown the mince. Once all the meat is completely browned, add the onion, carrot and celery and cook over a medium heat for about 10 minutes.

3. Add the garlic, cinnamon and rosemary and stir through, then add the chopped tomatoes and season with a little salt and pepper.

4. Bring to the boil then turn the heat right down, cover the pan with a lid and leave to simmer gently for about 10 minutes.

5. Meanwhile, cook the sweet potato in a large saucepan of boiling water until soft, then drain and leave to stand for a few minutes. Transfer to a large bowl, mash thoroughly with the Greek yogurt and a little salt and black pepper.

6. To bring it all together, pour the meat into an ovenproof dish, spoon on the mashed sweet potato and spread out evenly, then place in the oven to cook for about 40 to 45 minutes.

Chicken Nuggets with a Twist

Paired with sweet potato chips, you have no need to crave takeaways anymore!

1 free-range egg

100ml whole milk

2 tbsp Cajun spice mix

80g rolled oats

400g chicken breasts, cut
   into strips

1 tsp coconut oil, for frying

Green salad, to serve

Sweet potato fries, to serve

SERVES 2

1. In a small bowl, mix the egg and milk until completely combined.

2. In a separate dish, mix the Cajun spice with the oats until combined.

3. Using your hands, take each individual chicken strip and coat it in the egg mixture first, followed by the oats, and then leave to stand on a plate.

4. Once all coated, heat the coconut oil in a non-stick frying pan and fry the chicken strips until cooked through and crispy.

5. Serve with a green salad and sweet potato fries for the perfect evening meal.

Cauliflower Rice Tabbouleh with Fried Halloumi

A lovely light meal that is great for sharing.

1 cauliflower

50g fresh flat-leaf parsley, chopped

50g fresh mint, chopped

200g cherry tomatoes, halved and quartered

3 spring onions, thinly sliced

½ tsp coconut oil, for frying

200g halloumi, cut into thick slices

juice of 1 lemon

2 tbsp extra virgin olive oil

sea salt and freshly ground black pepper

SERVES 2

1. To make the cauliflower rice, first remove the core and the stalks from the cauliflower and blitz the cauliflower florets in a food processor until they resemble rice.

2. Place the cauliflower in a heatproof dish, and cover with clingfilm, ensuring you pierce a few holes into the film, then microwave for 6 to 7 minutes.

3. Remove from the microwave, remove the clingfilm and leave to stand for a few minutes before stirring through the parsley, mint, tomato and spring onion.

4. To fry the halloumi, heat the coconut oil in a frying pan, place the slices in the pan and cook over a medium to high heat for 1 to 2 minutes on each side.

5. Once slightly browned, place the halloumi onto the cauliflower rice tabbouleh and dress with the lemon juice, olive oil and a pinch of salt and pepper.

Homemade Turkey Burgers with Spicy Salsa and Guacamole

These are super easy to make and a delicious alternative to frozen or takeaway burgers. They are really healthy and great to serve to the kids too. Perfect for all the family.

FOR THE BURGERS

400g lean turkey mince

1/2 red onion, very finely
   chopped

1 garlic clove, crushed

1 tsp chopped fresh coriander

1 free-range egg yolk

coconut oil, for frying

sea salt and freshly ground
   black pepper

FOR THE SALSA

1/2 garlic clove, crushed

1/4 red onion, finely diced

coconut oil, for frying

100g tinned chopped tomatoes

1/2 tsp chilli flakes

FOR THE GUACAMOLE

1 large ripe avocado, halved
   and stone removed

juice of 1/2 lime

1 large ripe tomato, finely
   chopped

1/2 tbsp chopped fresh
   coriander

1 red chilli, deseeded and
   finely chopped

sea salt and freshly ground
   black pepper

SERVES 4

1. Place the turkey mince, red onion, garlic, coriander, egg yolk and a pinch of salt and pepper in a large mixing bowl and mix all the ingredients until completely combined. Using your hands, shape the mixture into 4 patties of equal size.

2. Next, in a small frying pan, make the salsa by heating your garlic and red onion in a little coconut oil before adding the chopped tomatoes and chilli flakes. Leave to simmer gently for about 5 minutes.

3. To make the guacamole, mash the avocado using a fork and then mix through the lime juice, tomato, coriander, chilli and a pinch of salt and pepper.

4. To cook the burgers, heat a small amount of coconut oil in a non-stick frying pan and place the patties in to fry, pressing them down gently with a spatula until they are cooked through and slightly browned on each side.

5. Serve the burgers topped with a tablespoon of guacamole, some fresh greens and a teaspoon of spicy salsa.

Health
is the
greatest
wealth

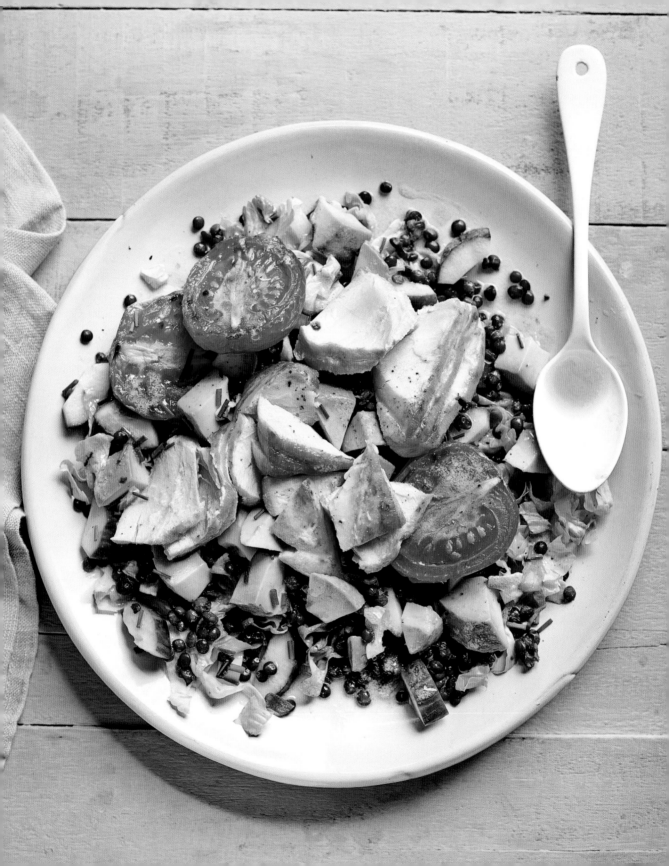

Salmon, Avocado and Balsamic Tomatoes with Puy Lentils and a Citrus Dressing

A multi-textured dish that is delicious hot or cold.

3-4 plum tomatoes, halved

2 tsp extra virgin olive oil

50ml balsamic vinegar

2 salmon fillets

1 baby gem lettuce, shredded

½ cucumber, halved, deseeded
   and cut into chunks

1 ripe avocado, stone removed
   and cut into small chunks

250g puy lentils, cooked

1 tsp chopped fresh chives

sea salt and freshly ground
   black pepper

FOR THE DRESSING

2 tbsp lemon juice

1 tsp Dijon mustard

2 tbsp cider vinegar

2 tbsp extra virgin olive oil

SERVES 2

1. Preheat the grill.

2. Place the tomatoes in a foil-lined roasting dish, season well with salt and pepper and then drizzle with olive oil and balsamic vinegar. Place them under the grill and cook until slightly browned on top. Remove and scrunch up the foil aound the tomatoes to keep them warm.

3. Season the salmon fillets then place under the hot grill for about 5 minutes, or until they are cooked.

4. Assemble the shredded baby gem lettuce, cucumber and avocado on a serving dish and scatter over the puy lentils and chives.

5. Once the salmon is cooked, remove the skin, flake the salmon onto the salad and top with the tomatoes.

6. Combine the dressing ingredients and drizzle over the finished salad.

Pan-fried Sea Bass with Miso, Lemon and Thyme-glazed Roasties

A tangy dish full of zing. The thyme adds deep flavour and the roasties give real crunch.

2 tbsp sweet white miso

juice of 1 lemon

2 tbsp coconut oil, melted

1 garlic clove, crushed

2 large carrots, cut into
    chunks

2 sweet potatoes, peeled and
    cut into chunks

2 large parsnips, cut into
    chunks

1 handful of fresh thyme

2 sea bass fillets

coconut oil, for frying

sea salt and freshly ground
    black pepper

SERVES 2

1. Preheat the oven to 200°C/400°F/Gas Mark 6.

2. In a mixing bowl, combine the miso paste, lemon juice, melted coconut oil and crushed garlic and stir well.

3. Lay the vegetables in a roasting dish, drizzle the miso glaze over the veg, then give the vegetables a good toss so that they are all coated.

4. Scatter the fresh thyme over the veg and a small sprinkling of sea salt then place into the hot oven for about 45 minutes.

5. When the vegetables are almost ready, prepare the sea bass by scoring the skin of the fillets with a sharp knife five or six times. Season with a little salt and pepper.

6. Heat a little coconut oil in a frying pan and place the sea bass in the pan, skin side down, to fry over a medium heat until the skin is crisp and brown. Flip over and cook for a further 2 minutes.

7. Lay a generous helping of roasted vegetables on a plate, top with the cooked sea bass and serve.

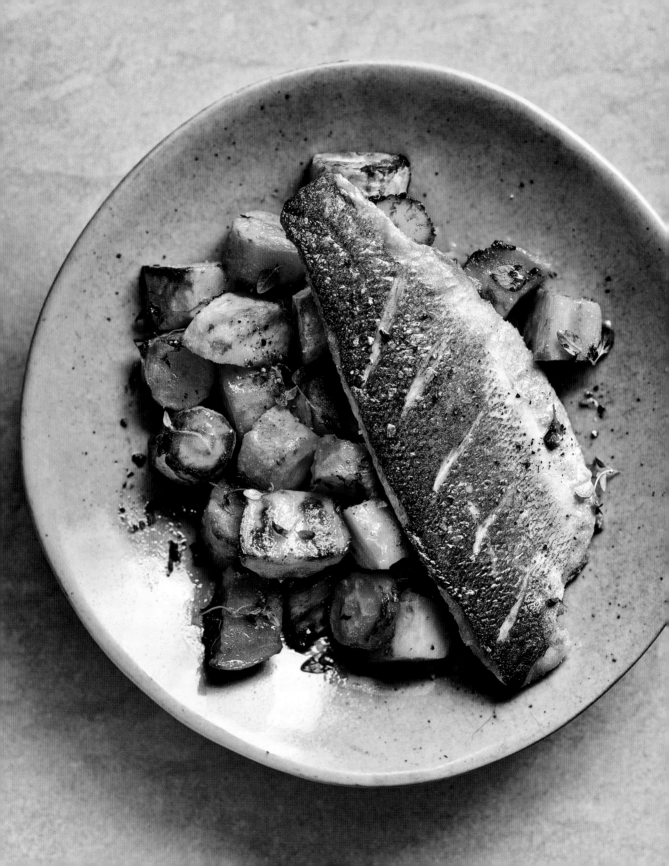

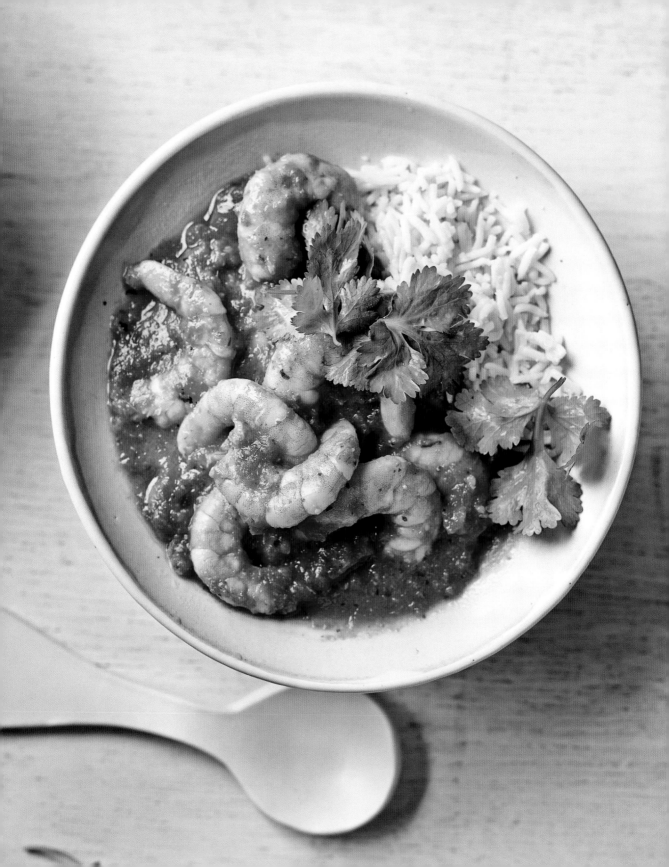

Prawn Masala

A healthy yet luxurious alternative to dialling for a takeaway, this is a tasty curry full of flavour.

FOR THE MASALA

½ tsp chilli flakes

1 tsp ground cumin

½ tsp ground turmeric

1 tsp ground coriander

freshly ground black pepper

1 onion, finely chopped

1 garlic clove, crushed

5cm chunk of fresh ginger, grated

1 small handful of fresh coriander, plus extra to serve

coconut oil

400g tinned chopped tomatoes

150g raw king prawns, peeled

juice of 1 lemon, to serve

cooked rice, to serve (optional)

SERVES 2

1. Mix all the masala spices together.

2. Mix together the onion, garlic, ginger and two-thirds of the coriander and blend in a food processor until smooth.

3. Fry this paste in a little coconut oil for about 1 minute before adding the masala spices. Fry for a few more minutes, then add the chopped tomatoes, bring to a simmer, and cook for a further 10 minutes until thickened. You may want to add a splash of water if it becomes too dry.

4. Stir your prawns into the mixture and cook until pink.

5. Serve with rice, if desired, a scattering of fresh coriander and a squeeze of lemon.

Grilled Tuna Steaks with Roasted Red Pepper Sauce and Broccoli Rice

A super-healthy, protein-packed plate of goodness.

2 red peppers, deseeded and halved

coconut oil, for greasing and frying

200g tomato passata

1 garlic clove, crushed

½ red onion, very finely diced

1 small handful of fresh basil, chopped

2 tuna steaks

FOR THE BROCCOLI RICE

1 whole head broccoli

pinch of garlic salt

SERVES 2

1. Preheat the grill.

2. Using your hands, rub the peppers with a little coconut oil, then lay on a foil-lined tray and place under the grill for about 10 minutes until blackened.

3. Once cooked, leave to stand and cool for a few minutes, then remove the skins and blitz the peppers in a food processor until smooth, adding a little of the passata to loosen.

4. In a frying pan, heat a little coconut oil then add the garlic and red onion and fry for a few minutes.

5. Add the red pepper and passata and simmer gently for about 10 minutes. Stir in the basil leaves.

6. Meanwhile, cut the core and stalks from the broccoli head and pulse the broccoli heads in a food processor until they resemble rice. Place this into a heatproof dish and cover with clingfilm, ensuring you pierce the film to create a few air holes. Season with a little garlic salt, stir through, and microwave on high for about 7 minutes.

7. In a frying pan, heat a little coconut oil and fry the tuna steaks for about 3 minutes on each side.

8. Plate up a generous helping of broccoli rice, top with a sliced tuna steak and finish with a helping of red pepper sauce.

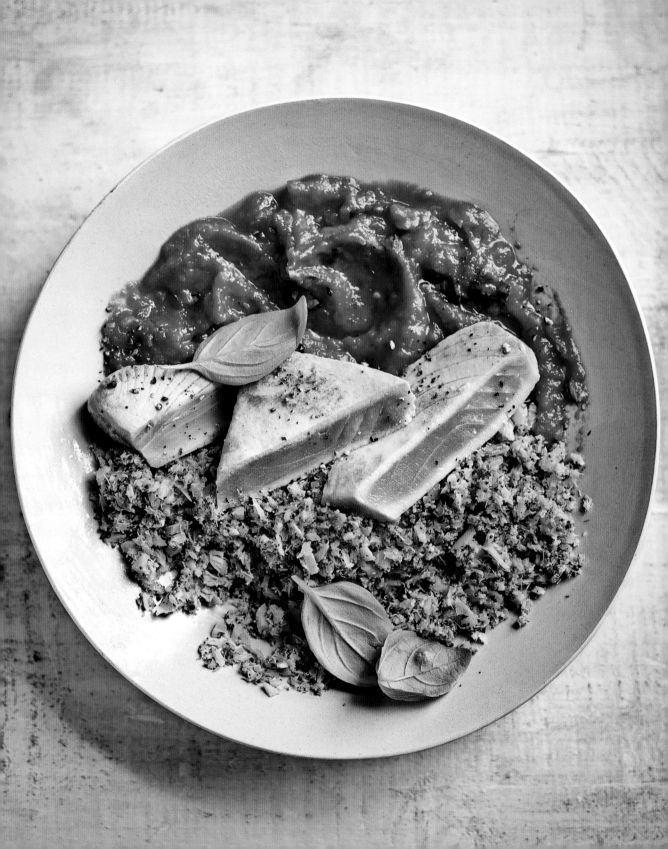

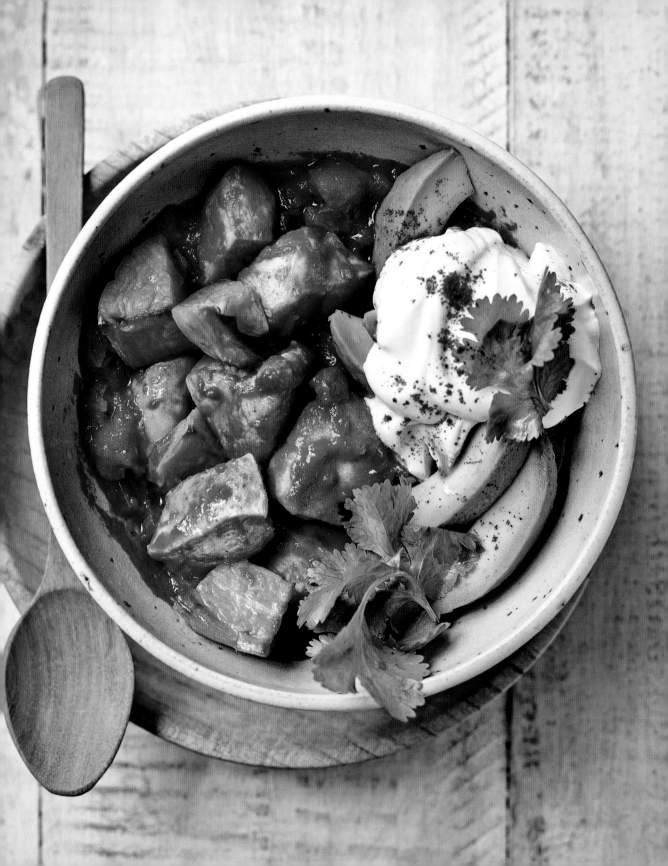

Mexican-style Spicy Sweet Potato and Chicken Bowl

A one-pot evening meal with minimum fuss and maximum taste.

2 sweet potatoes, peeled and
    chopped into chunks

coconut oil, for greasing and
    frying

1 garlic clove, crushed

1 red onion, finely diced

200g skinless chicken breast,
    cut into chunks

1 tsp paprika, plus extra for
    sprinkling

200g tinned chopped tomatoes

1 ripe avocado, stone removed
    and flesh cut into chunks

2 tbsp sour cream

1 small handful of fresh
    coriander

sea salt and freshly ground
    black pepper

SERVES 2

1. Preheat the oven to 200°C/400°F/Gas Mark 6.

2. Massage the sweet potato chunks with a little coconut oil, season well and then place onto a foil-lined tray. Bake in the oven for about 35 minutes.

3. Meanwhile, heat a small amount of coconut oil in a frying pan, add the garlic and red onion and fry gently until slightly softened. Add the chicken breast chunks, lightly season with paprika and a pinch of salt and pepper and brown the chicken for a few minutes.

4. Add the chopped tomatoes, then leave to simmer for 20 minutes until thickened.

5. Once the sweet potato is cooked, add to the pan and stir through.

6. Plate up, add the avocado, sour cream and sprinkle with fresh coriander paprika and serve.

SNACKS

The most important thing to remember is that this isn't a diet, so snacks are very much allowed. To me they are a vital part of what I consume every day.

A healthy snack is the perfect pick-me-up after a busy morning or afternoon and can carry you through to lunch after a morning workout or be the vital blast of energy needed before evening exercise.

By prepping these delicious snacks in advance, you will avoid the sugary, unhealthy treats often lying around the office or found at the back of the cupboard. After all your hard work preparing three main meals, it is so easy to fall down when it comes to snacking – proper planning will ensure that you stay focused and committed without giving in to temptation.

Kale Dip with Raw Veg Dippers

A delicious dip to get your supply of leafy greens.

50g kale, tough stalks
    removed

150g Greek yogurt

½ tsp garlic paste

squeeze of lemon juice

pinch of chilli flakes

2 carrots, cut into batons

2 celery sticks, cut into
    batons

sea salt and freshly ground
    black pepper

SERVES 2

1. Steam the kale for about 4 minutes or use a microwave. Transfer to a sieve and rinse under cold water for 2 to 3 minutes until cooled. Then, using a fork or spoon, try to remove as much excess liquid as possible.

2. Put the kale, Greek yogurt and garlic paste, as well as a good grind of pepper and salt, into a blender and blitz until smooth. Add the lemon juice and chilli flakes and enjoy with the pre-prepped vegetable batons.

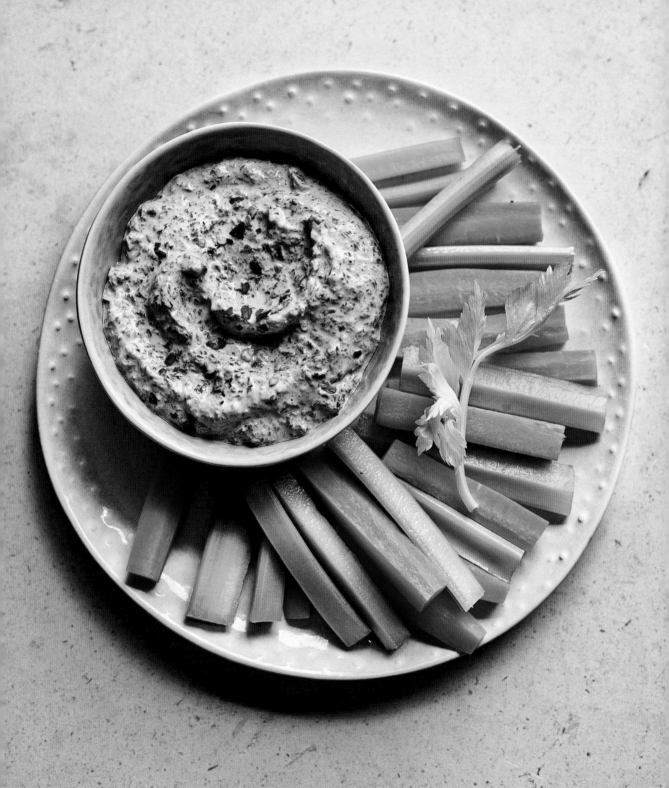

Courgette Hummus on Rice Cakes

Courgettes have made a real comeback in the healthy foodie world and I love this recipe for a fresh twist on the classic hummus.

2 courgettes

1 tbsp coconut oil

80g tahini

2-3 ice cubes

1 garlic clove, crushed

juice of ½ lemon, plus extra to finish

1 tsp smoked paprika

6 rice cakes, to serve

sea salt

SERVES 2

1. Roughly chop the courgettes and place in a food processor with the coconut oil, tahini, ice cubes, garlic, lemon juice, a pinch of salt and half of the paprika and pulse until completely smooth.

2. Serve in a dish and top with the remaining paprika and an extra squeeze of lemon juice, then spread onto rice cakes.

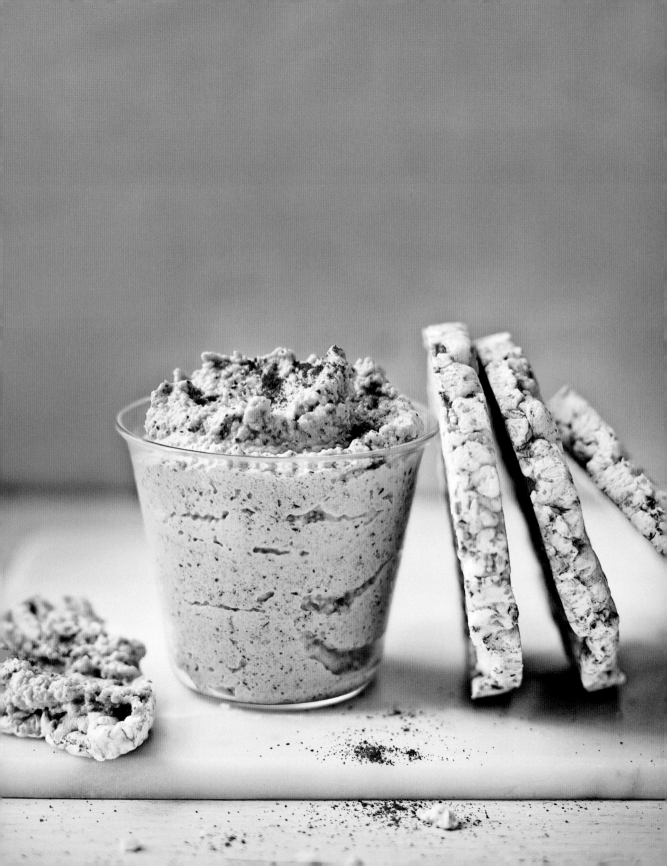

Superfood Chocolate Protein Smoothie

2 frozen bananas

2 tbsp cacao powder

½ tsp vanilla powder

1 tbsp peanut butter or other
   nut butter

1 scoop of whey protein
   powder (chocolate flavour
   if possible, but natural or
   vanilla will work too)

100ml water

SERVES 2

The most delicious post-workout chocolatey hit. Packed full of goodness, this definitely trumps any sugar-loaded chocolate bar.

Place everything in a blender and blitz until fully combined and smooth.

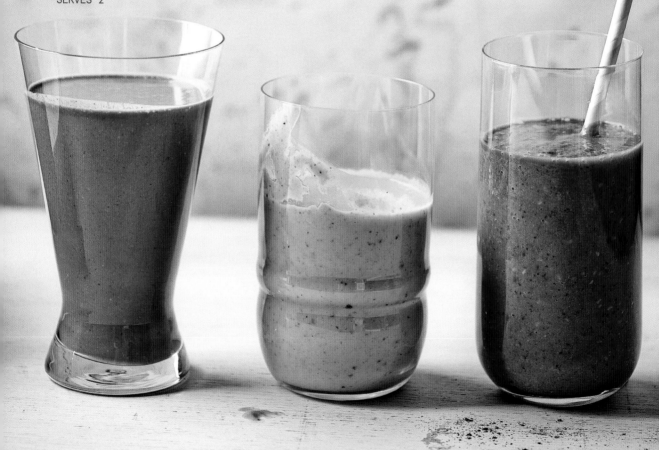

Berry Blast Smoothie

Berries are low in fructose and packed full of antioxidants, providing you with a delicious and light snack that will leave you feeling energized!

½ frozen banana

1 tbsp Greek yogurt

½ tsp ground cinnamon

100g raspberries

100g blueberries

Handful of spinach

100ml almond milk

SERVES 2

Blend all the ingredients in a blender or smoothie maker until fully combined and enjoy.

Cashew and Goji Berry Energy Balls

Prepped in advance, these are great for a snack-on-the-go to fuel a busy day!

3 tbsp chopped unsalted
  cashew nuts

3 tbsp goji berries, roughly
  chopped

2 tbsp sunflower seeds

2 tbsp agave nectar

3 tbsp milled flaxseed

1 tbsp desiccated coconut

MAKES ABOUT 12 BALLS

1. Pulse all the ingredients except the coconut in a blender until well combined.

2. Using your hands, form about 12 small balls with the mixture and cover in a light coating of desiccated coconut. Transfer to a plate to chill for about 30 minutes.

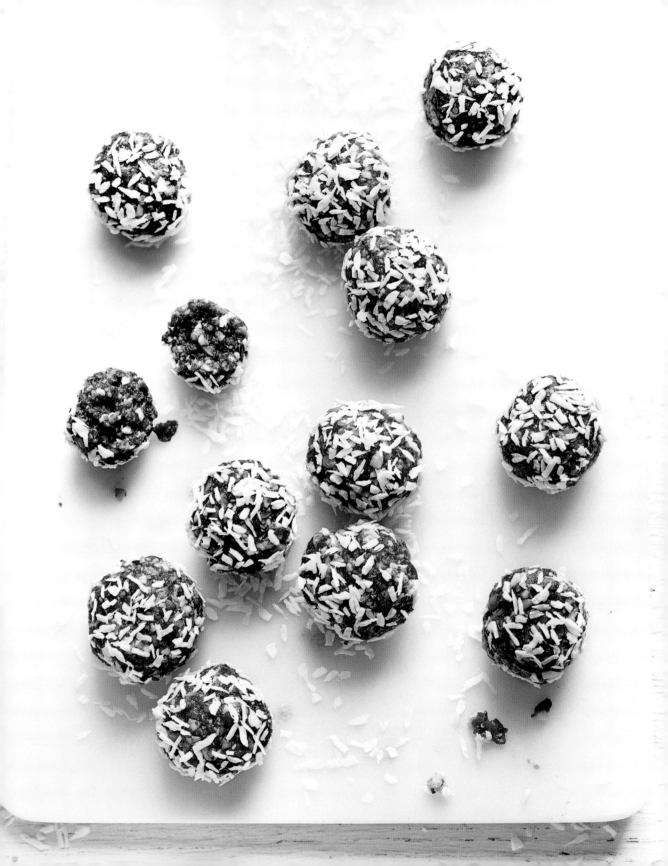

EXERCISE

There is no right or wrong way to get active and exercise. You just have to find something you love, do it and stick to it!

Finding your favourite form of exercise, be it cycling, jogging or heading to classes at your local gym, will ensure that you're much more likely to keep at it and maintain motivation.

I think that's one of the things that really clicked with me when I began my journey. I started going to the gym and suddenly found a way of exercising that I enjoyed. I began to feel confident and so started burning calories in a way that didn't make it feel like a horrible chore. Exercise stopped being that thing I needed to do but couldn't find the motivation for, and became the thing that framed my day and made me feel great. I knew it was the means to the end – the thing that would get me the body and mindset I wanted.

I have a lot of people asking me on Instagram how I got the shape I have, so this book is about sharing that message with you. There is no smoke and mirrors here; I am going to be very honest about the hard work I put in. I want to provide a practical way of helping you understand how you can combine the right diet and the right training programme and how quickly it can become second nature.

I was unhappy with my body, that's why I made the change, but I wanted something straightforward that I could commit to and enjoy. That's what this book is for me. I wasn't proud of how I looked or felt, I wasn't happy with how I was performing in my degree, so I took the leap and turned my life around.

I am now at a healthy weight and have achieved the body I dreamed of. I took control and there is no better feeling.

Although, as the saying goes, 'You can't out-train a bad diet,' exercise is what will help you create a lean and defined physique.

In this book I'm sharing with you some of my favourite exercises from the gym that you can do in the comfort of your own home. What I want to help you do is break a sweat, feel confident with the exercises, and start to see real muscle definition through working each muscle group individually.

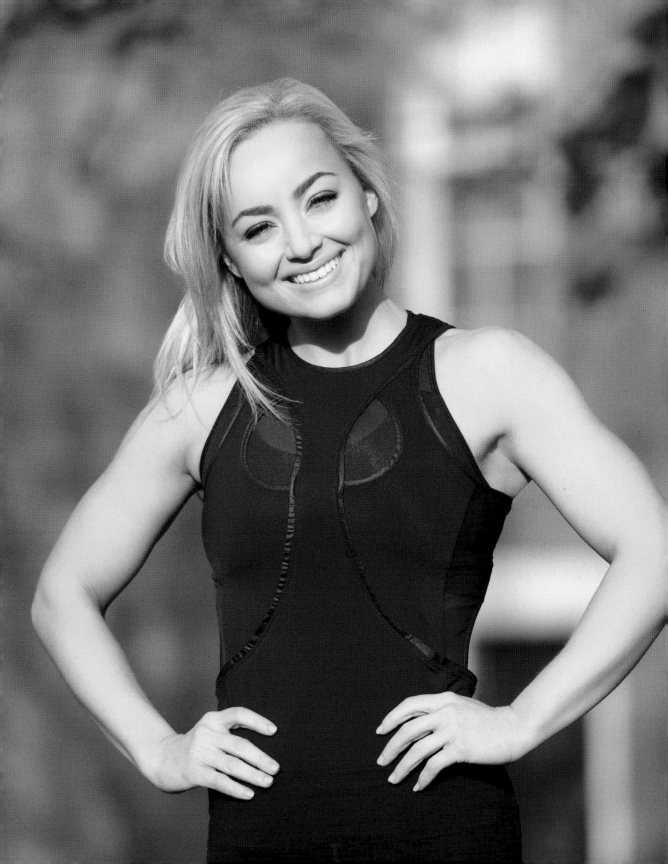

GETTING STARTED

It's important to always do a warm-up before exercising, to increase muscle temperature and avoid injury. Warming-up can be as simple as jogging on the spot or some jumping jacks – anything to increase your heart rate and get your blood circulating to prepare your muscles for a workout!

It's also important to remember to keep hydrated throughout your workout by drinking plenty of water.

EXERCISE

The main aim in this book is for me to show you that exercise doesn't have to be a chore. It is an easy habit to make and one you don't need to break.

Exercise is a funny thing really. From a young age it's ingrained in us that keeping fit is not something to be enjoyed. We all go through our school days skipping games and PE, moaning about cold and muddy cross-country runs, and it is easy to take that attitude with us into adult life. Exercise then becomes something to be suffered if we need to lose a few pounds for a bikini holiday or after the Christmas excess. It becomes a short-term means to a short-term end, rather than being something to enjoy, celebrate and implement for the long term. It becomes about controlling weight rather than loving our bodies and we spend more time talking about why we can't do it than we do actually getting on with it!

We all know the drill. We say we want to get in shape, and that we need to tone up, but then the problem is lack of time. How many times have we all uttered the words, 'I wish I had time to go to the gym,' and then sat on the sofa with another glass of wine or bar of chocolate, thinking, 'There's no point now, I've done the damage.' Exercise needs to be built into your everyday life if there is any chance of doing it regularly – and doing it regularly is the only way you will see permanent results.

The first thing you need to do is find exercises that you like.

This is KEY – you will not stick to any form of exercise if you can't stand the thought of doing it! I am a great believer that you achieve far more physically and mentally by doing 20 minutes of something you love, rather than spending an hour in the gym wandering around using machines you can't work and that you hate. Even if the chosen exercise is a brisk 20-minute walk with the dog, buggy or the iPod, that's fantastic because it is SOMETHING!

The exercises that follow are ideal for people who find the gym boring, expensive, daunting or simply pointless. It is the perfect kind of exercise for people who are short on time, like to be challenged and want real results. The programme doesn't require a fancy gym membership, a personal trainer, or loads of equipment you will use a few times and then watch gather dust in the upstairs cupboard.

All you need is YOU, a commitment to getting fit and a determination to make a change for life.

The sessions that follow last 20 to 30 minutes and are broken down by body area, allowing you to individually target each muscle group.

The aim with the exercises is that you will train four to five times a week for 20 to 30 minutes at a time.

This is at the heart of why high-impact exercise works, but it is also because I believe this is a time frame that is achievable and can be woven into a busy day for the average person. If you over-complicate it or make your session last too long, you are guaranteed to stop due to lack of time. Exercise is the easiest thing to banish from a fraught or hectic day when, ironically, it is often the thing that will make you feel instantly better and relieve any stress.

Just as the recipe section isn't about drinking juice or restricting your calories, this fitness section isn't about exercising twice a day for seven days to dramatically lose weight. It is about long-term healthy living. This is not a quick-fix weight-loss programme that ends up with the weight being all be piled back on as soon as you go back to your 'normal' way of living. This is about creating a new 'normal' that becomes permanent.

However, to reach your goal you must also follow a proper diet. Diet is the crux of the entire plan and is the foundation of a healthy body and a healthy mind – it is 60 per cent of what you need to whip yourself into shape.

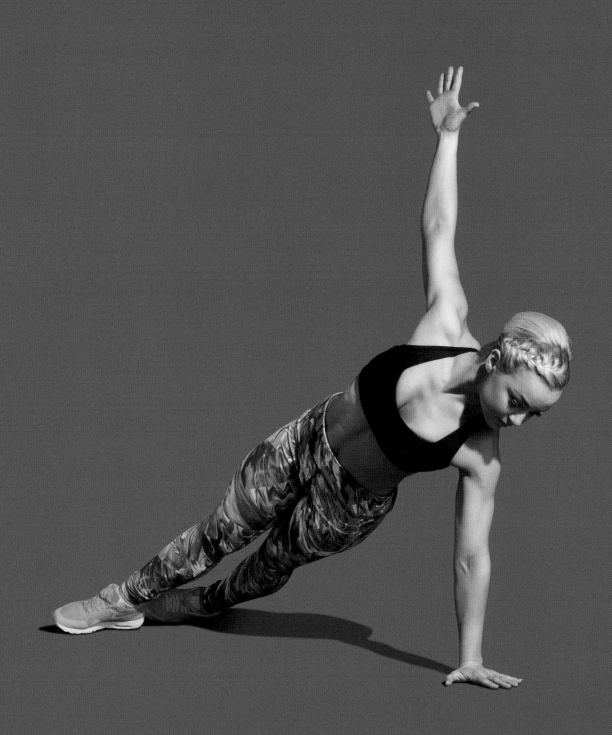

GET MOVING. GET ENERGIZED.

Optional equipment to be used in either the gym or at home:

A SWISS BALL | A BAR BELL

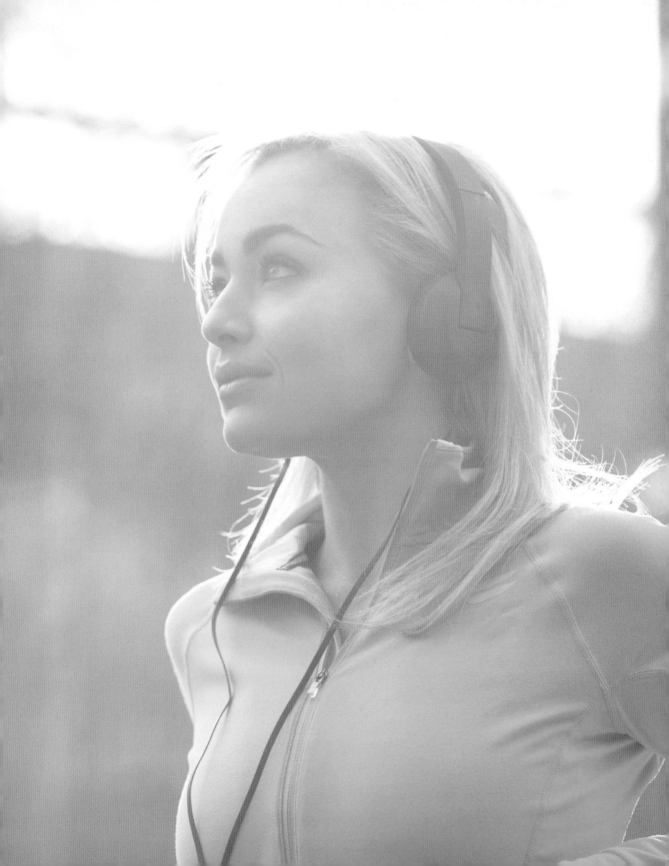

1

Legs

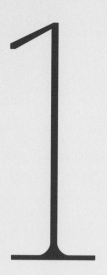

1 Legs

Designed to train your legs and your mind and to fire up your thighs, glutes and core.

Equipment needed:

A SWISS BALL

A BAR BELL

A BOX OR
STURDY CHAIR

A KETTLE BELL

WARM-UP

Begin your warm-up with some mobilization and activation of the leg and gluteus muscles to increase the muscle temperature and avoid injury.

Walking Lunges

REPS: 3X20 (30-second rest between each set)

· Stand up straight, with your feet together, placing your hands by your sides. Make sure that you push your chest out and have your shoulders back.

· With your feet still together, step one foot forward into a lunge position.

· Bend both knees to around a 90-degree angle. As you place your foot on the floor in front of you, make sure your knee is in line with your ankle. The back knee should also be just above the floor.

· Make sure your knees don't roll in or out, then drive and push up out of the lunge until both feet meet together again.

· Repeat on other leg.

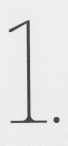

1.

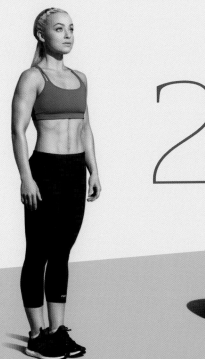

2.

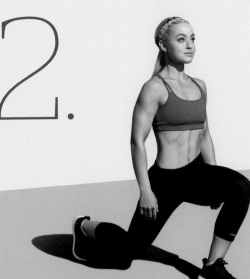

Feet-elevated Glute Bridges

REPS: 3X15 (30-second rest between each set)

EXERCISE

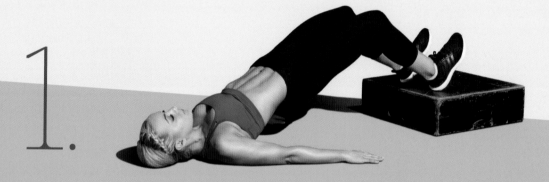

1.

· Place both heels on an elevated platform (about a foot off the floor) so that your toes are pointing upwards.

· Place the top of your back on the floor, then drive your hips upwards to create a bridge position, then lower down again.

· Make sure you engage your glutes and don't roll your knees in or out.

· Once you're feeling warm and energized, begin your booty workout.

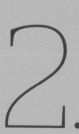

2.

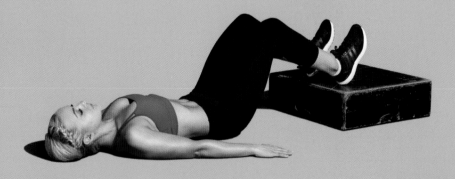

Basic Squat

REPS: 4X12 (30-second - 1-minute rest between each set)

- Step your feet slightly wider than hip width apart and have your feet at a comfortable angle, either with toes facing forwards or slightly turned out.

- Keep your chest up. Perhaps aid this by crossing your arms onto your chest.

- Breathe in and lower yourself down (as if you were going to sit on a chair), without your knees rolling in or out and ensuring your heels stay on the ground.

- Bend at both the hips and the knees.

- Once at the bottom of your squat, engage your glutes and legs and drive back up to standing position, avoiding fully locking out the knees or hyperextending (your upper legs should be parallel with the floor and your back should be between a 45- and 90-degree angle to your hips).

147

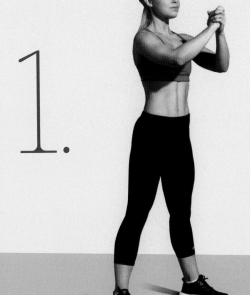

1.

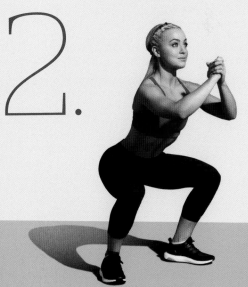

2.

Step-ups

REPS: 4X12 (Twice with right leg leading, twice with left leg leading. 30-second – 1-minute rest between each)

· Place a sturdy chair, stair or box in front of you.

· Step up and place your whole foot (not just the toes) on the surface, making sure your knee does not extend over your toes.

· As you place your foot on the platform, push right through the heel so that you really work your glutes (rather than pushing up on your toes or the front of the foot).

· On the push up, drive through one leg, then bring the other up to meet it.

· Step back down with the first leg, then repeat with the opposite leg leading.

148

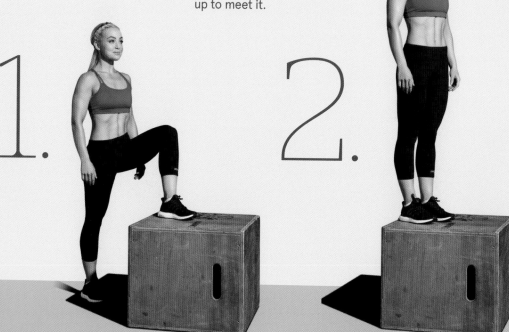

1.

2.

Wide Sumo Squats with 2-second Pulse at the Bottom

REPS: 4X12 (30-second - 1-minute rest between each set)

· Take your feet into a similar stance to the basic squat, but with your feet slightly wider, and the toes facing slightly out.

· Keep your chest up and bend at the knee as if you were going to sit on a chair.

· Look straight ahead and make sure your knees are bent and in line with your hips.

· Continue bending your knees until your upper legs are parallel with the floor, ensuring that your back remains

between a 45- and 90- degree angle to your hips.

· Drive up through the legs and glutes to full extension, making sure you don't roll or lock out the knees.

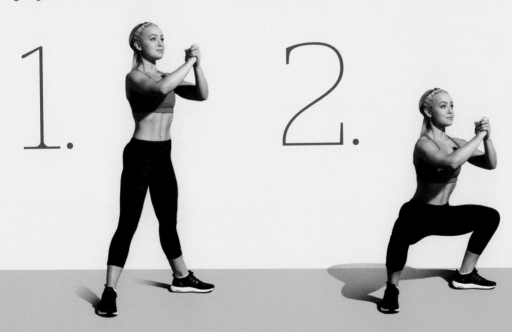

1.

2.

Tuck Jump to Squat

REPS: 4X10 (30-second - 1-minute rest between each set)

- Place both feet on the floor wider than shoulder width, with your feet facing forward.

- In a jumping motion, bring your knees up to your chest in a tuck jump.

- As you land, place your feet slightly wider than hip width apart and assume the squat position. Ensure you keep your chest up and your knees don't roll in or out.

- When you've completed your squat, bring your feet back in together to prepare to tuck jump again and repeat.

150

EXERCISE

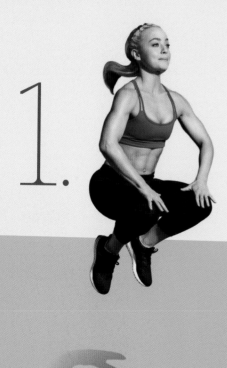

1.

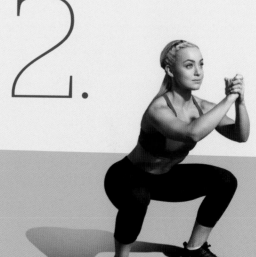

2.

Bulgarian Split Squat

REPS: 4X12 EACH SIDE (30-second - 1-minute rest between each set)

· This is similar to a classic lunge.

· Rest your back foot on a sturdy chair, stair or box and step the front foot out so you are able to achieve a deep lunge.

· Keep your chest up and ensure your knees don't roll in or out.

· Bend to the bottom of your lunge, then drive up to full extension.

· Repeat for the other leg.

151

EXERCISE

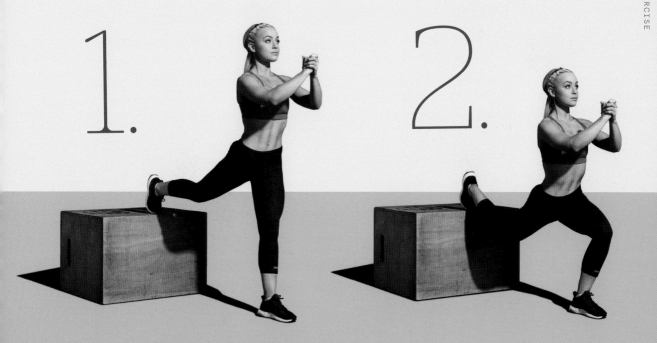

Feet-elevated Glute Bridges

REPS: 4X15 (30-second - 1-minute rest between each set)

EXERCISE

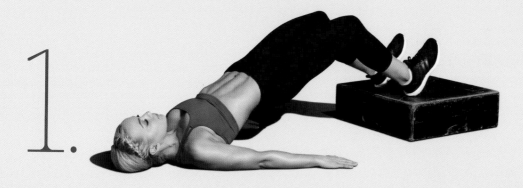

1.

· Repeating from the warm-up section, place both heels on an elevated platform (about a foot off the floor) so that your toes are pointing upwards.

· Place the top of your back on the floor, then drive your hips upwards to create a bridge position, then lower down again.

· Make sure you engage your glutes and don't roll your knees in or out.

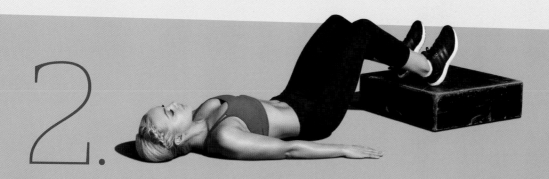

2.

Jumping Toe Taps

REPS: 20X4 (1-minute rest between each set)

- Using a sturdy chair, stair or box, tap one toe on the chair, then quickly tap the other.

- Use your arms to power you and add speed.

- Keep your chest up.

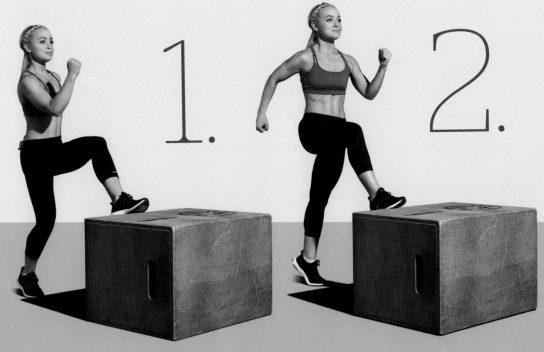

1.

2.

8-10 Squat Jumps

· This is similar to your basic squat, but this time you're going to jump as you come back up.

· Keeping your chest up and your knees sturdy, drive up through your legs and glutes, jumping up as you come out of your squat.

154

EXERCISE

1.

2.

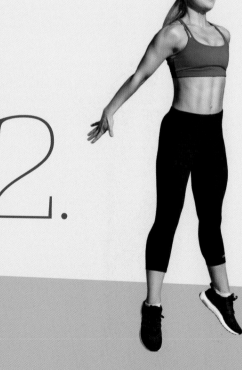

Wall-sit

STAY THERE AS LONG AS POSSIBLE – CHALLENGE YOURSELF

· Rest your back against a wall,
  then slide down so your knees
  are at a right angle, as if you
  were sitting on a chair.

· Hold for as long as possible.

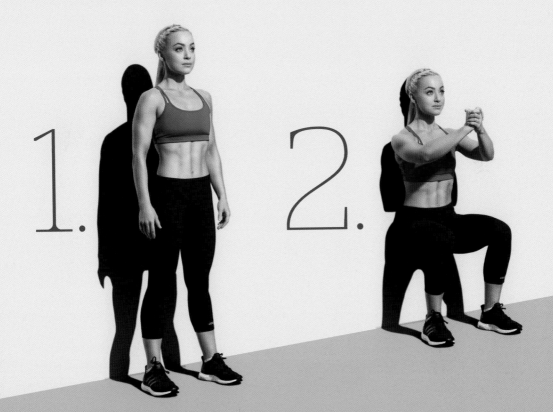

155

2

Upper Body
and Abs

2 Upper Body and Abs

EXERCISE

Designed to give you abs of steel and the perfect all-year-round bikini body.

Equipment needed:

A SWISS BALL

A BOX OR STURDY CHAIR

WARM-UP

Begin your warm-up with some mobilization and activation of the upper body, until you feel warm.

Full-body Press-ups

REPS : 3X8 (30-second - 1-minute rest between each set)

· Start with both hands on the floor, shoulder width apart.

· Take your arms to either side of your chest with your hands facing forwards.

· Keep your feet together behind you, resting on the balls of your feet.

· Bend at the elbow ensuring your entire body remains completely flat, so no dipping at the hips or through the back.

· Keep your back straight and use your core to stabilize through your abdominal muscles.

· Push through your chest and extend your arms to lift your body, then drive up to full extension.

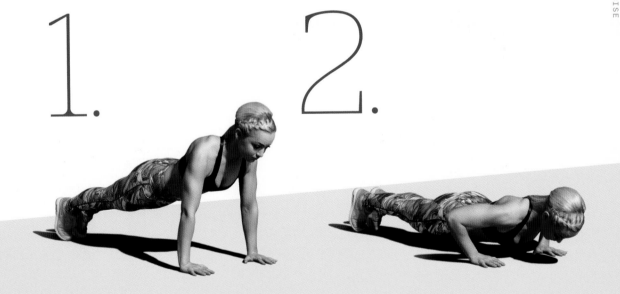

Mountain Climbers

REPS: 3X20 (30-second – 1-minute rest between each set)

· Start in push-up position with arms wider than your shoulders and put your body weight over your hands.

· Take your arms to either side of your chest with your hands facing forwards.

· Bend at the elbow ensuring your entire body remains completely flat, so no dipping at the hips or through the back. Extend your arms so you make a flat plank.

· Keeping one foot on the floor, bring one knee into your chest, alternating as if running at a quick pace, ensuring your core remains solid and there is no dipping through the pelvis or back.

· Increase your speed, as if you are running on your hands.

160

EXERCISE

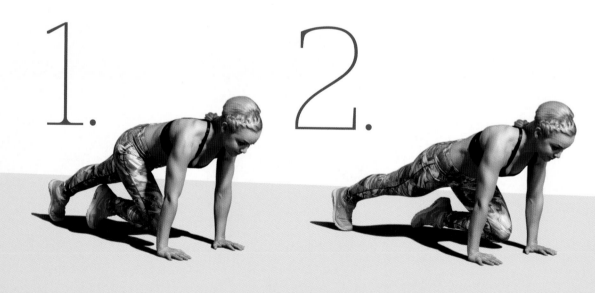

Neutral-stance Press-ups

REPS: 4X10 (1-minute rest between each set)

• As per the warm-up on page
  159, repeat your press-ups.

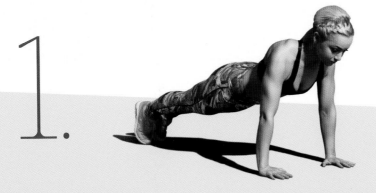

1.

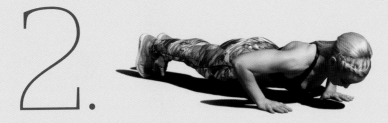

2.

Star Twists

REPS: 4X20 (30-second - 1-minute rest between each set)

· Keep your arms at full extension as in your plank position.

· Open one arm out laterally, so your entire body faces one side.

· Keep your hips up and your core tight, your head in line, then repeat, opening up the opposite arm.

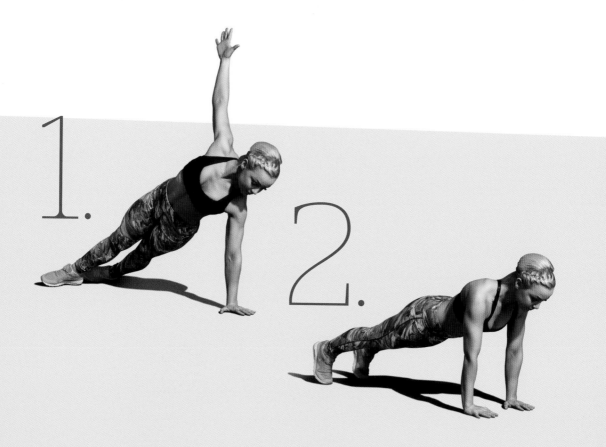

Wide-stance Press-ups

REPS: 4X10 (30-second - 1-minute rest between each set)

· Positioning for this one is the same as your neutral-stance press-ups, but this time take your hands wide.

· Your range of motion may not be as fast with this wider positioning, but still remember to keep your core tight and your head in line. Take these slowly to really feel the burn.

· Keep your back straight and stabilize through your core.

· Push through your chest and extend your arms to lift your body back into push-up position.

163

EXERCISE

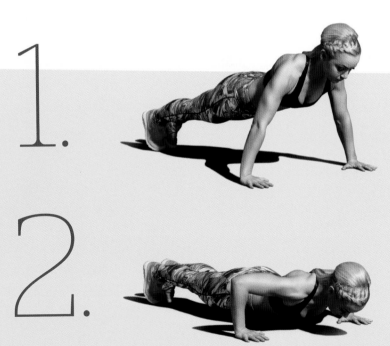

1.

2.

Hand Taps

REPS: 4X20 (30-second – 1-minute rest between each set)

· Once you have done your press-ups, extend your body into full plank position, ensuring your core is tight and your head is in line.

· While still in plank position, lift one hand off the floor and tap the other hand. Then repeat with the other hand.

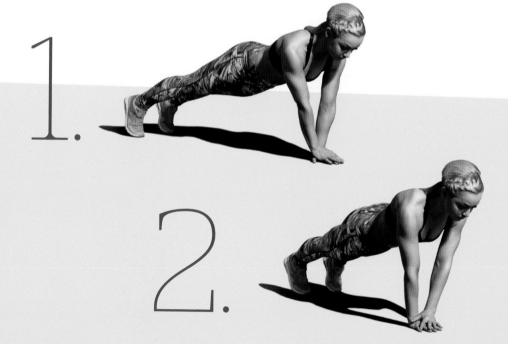

1.

2.

Arrow Press

REPS: 4X10 (30-second rest between each set)

· Bring your hands into a prayer position, then turn your hands so your fingers point forwards.

· Squeeze your hands together so there is definite tension in the arms.

· Keeping your hands pressed together, drive forwards and then return them slowly into your chest.

165

EXERCISE

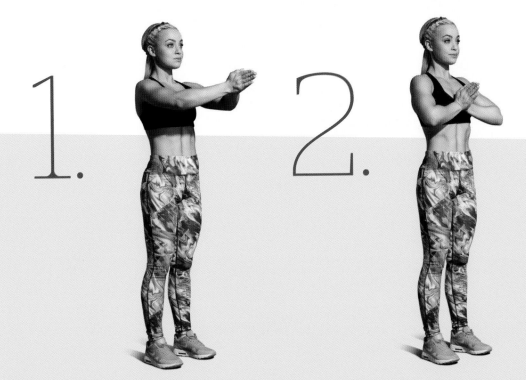

1.   2.

Tricep Dips

REPS: 4X10 (30-second rest between each set)

- Sit on the edge of a sturdy chair, stair or box and place your hands on either side of you with your hands pointing forwards. Your hands should be underneath your bum and approximately shoulder width apart.

- Edge off the chair so that your feet are either fully extended so you resemble a plank, or place them so your legs are at a right angle. This is your starting position.

- Bend at the elbows so you dip your body, creating a 90-degree angle with your hips.

- Drive up through the arms back to your initial position.

- Do not use your legs to help; all the activity should be through your core and the arms.

166

EXERCISE

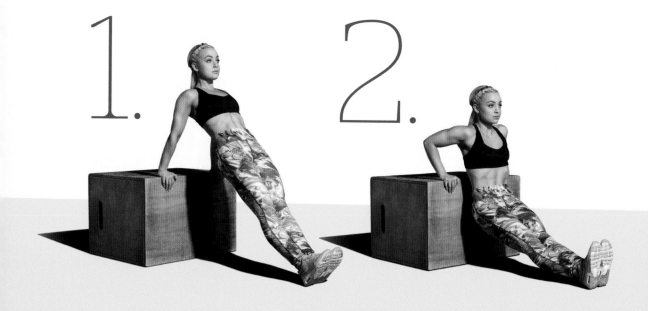

Tricep Kickbacks

REPS: 4X10 (20 each side, 30-second rest between each)

- Using any form of weight (either dumbbells, soup cans or any alternatives) bend at the hip so you are at a right angle.

- Bend both arms at the elbow.

- At a slight angle, extend your arms backwards to full extension.

- Be careful not to fully lock out the elbow.

- Return to original position.

167

EXERCISE

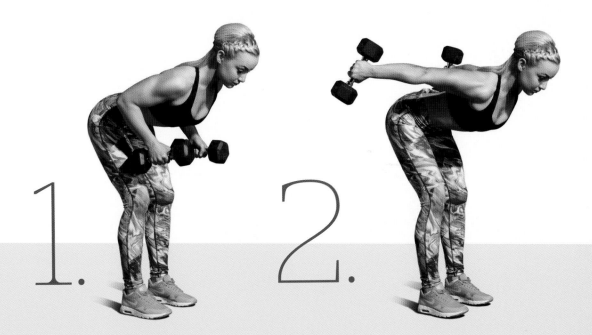

Diamond Press-ups

REPS: 3X5 (30-second rest between each set)

- Place your hands in a diamond position, so your index finger and thumb are together.

- Keeping your core tight and head in line, lower into your press-up, then drive up to full extension.

- Repeat as above.

1.

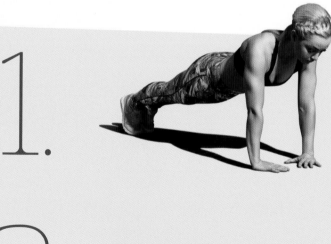

2.

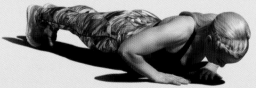

Plank

HOLD FOR AS LONG AS POSSIBLE - CHALLENGE YOURSELF

· Get into your plank position
  with your arms fully extended.

· Keep your feet together and
  your core tight so there is no
  dip in the pelvis or back.

· Hold for as long as possible.

1.

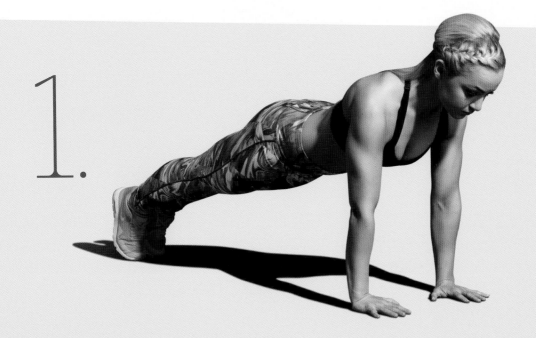

Lying-down Burpees

REPS: 8

· Lying flat face-down on the ground, place your arms stretched above your head.

· Press yourself up into a crouched position and jump upwards before crouching back down.

· Return to your original position with your arms stretched above your head.

1.

2.

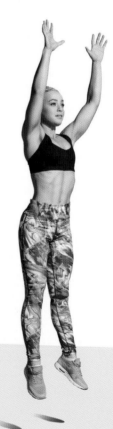

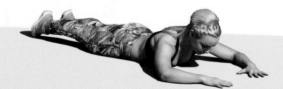

It doesn't matter how slowly you go as long as you do not stop

3

Legs and Abs

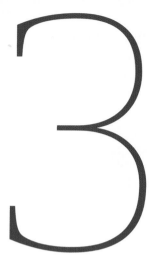

3

Legs and Abs

Designed to enhance the abdominal area and tone your legs.

Equipment needed:

A SWISS BALL | A BAR BELL | A KETTLE BELL

WARM-UP

Begin your warm-up with some mobilization and activation of the leg muscles.

Walking Lunges

REPS: 2X20 (10 each side, 30-second - 1-minute rest between each set)

- Stand up straight, with your feet together, placing your hands by your sides. Make sure that you push your chest out and have your shoulders back.

- With your feet still together, step one foot forward into a lunge position.

- Bend both knees at around 90 degrees. As you place your foot on the floor in front of you, make sure your knee is in line with your ankle. The back knee should also be just above the floor.

- Make sure your knees don't roll in or out, then drive and push up out of the lunge until both feet meet together again.

- Repeat on the other leg.

175

EXERCISE

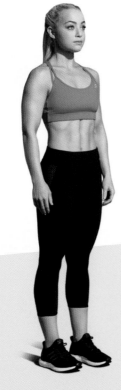

1.

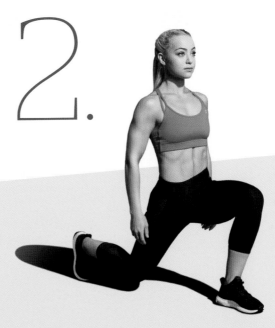

2.

Monster Walks

REPS: 20X2 (30-second - 1-minute rest between each set)

· Similar to walking lunges, except this time take your feet slightly wider so you can really open up your hips. Ensure your knees don't roll in or out. Keep your chest up and core tight.

· Once your muscles feel warm and energized, you can begin your workout.

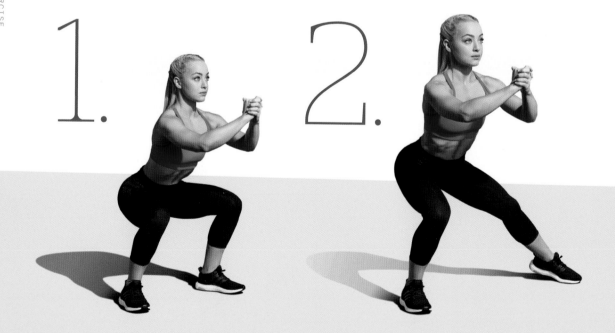

1. 2.

Basic Squat with 5-second Hold

REPS: 4X12 (30-seconds - 1-minute rest between each set)

· Exactly the same as your
  Basic Squat on page 147,
  but this time hold the bottom
  of your squat position for
  5 seconds before driving up
  to full extension.

177

EXERCISE

1.

2.

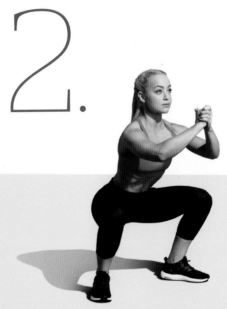

Kettle Bell Deadlift

REPS: 4X12 (1-minute rest between each set)

· Using a kettle bell, dumbbell or weight, bend at the hips keeping your back flat and your legs slightly soft but not too bent.

· Lower yourself down until you feel a pull on your hamstring.

· Using your legs and glutes, drive back up to your original position.

1.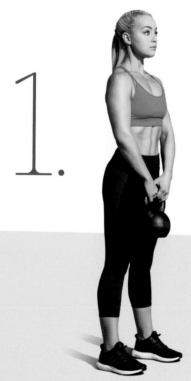

2.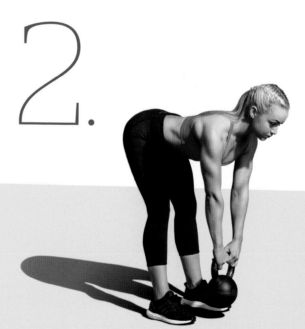

Sumo Squats with 2-second Hold at the Bottom

REPS: 4X12 (30-second – 1-minute rest between each set)

· Take your feet into a similar stance to the basic squat, but with your feet slightly wider, and the toes facing slightly out.

· Keep your chest up and bend at the knee as if you were going to sit on a chair.

· Look straight ahead and make sure your knees are bent and in line with your hips.

· Continue bending your knees until your upper legs are parallel with the floor, ensuring that your back remains between a 45- and 90-degree angle to your hips.

· Hold for 2 seconds, then drive up through the legs and glutes to full extension, making sure you don't roll or lock out the knees.

1.

2.

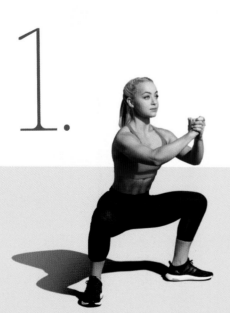
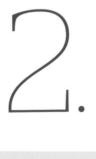
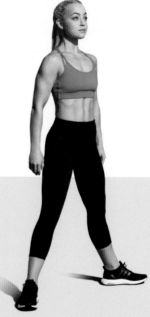

Walking Lunges with Pulse

REPS: 4X20 (30-second – 1-minute rest between each set)

· Stand up straight, with your feet together, placing your hands by your sides. Make sure that you push your chest out and have your shoulders back.

· With your feet still together, step one foot forward into a lunge position.

· Bend both knees to around a 90-degree angle. As you place your foot on the floor in front of you, make sure your knee is in line with your ankle. The back knee should also be just above the floor.

· Make sure your knees don't roll in or out, then drive and push up out of the lunge until both feet meet together again.

· Repeat on other leg.

180

EXERCISE

1.

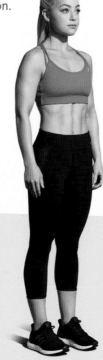

2.

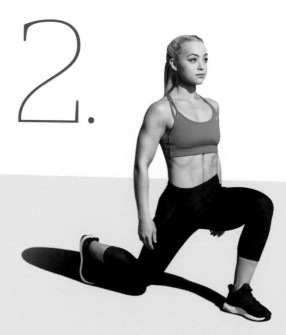

Feet-elevated Plank

REPS: 3X30 (30-second - 1-minute rest between each set)

· Place your feet on an elevated platform, about a foot off the floor.

· Get into your plank position, keeping your core tight and head in line.

· Ensure there is no dip in the pelvis or back. Hold the position for 30 seconds.

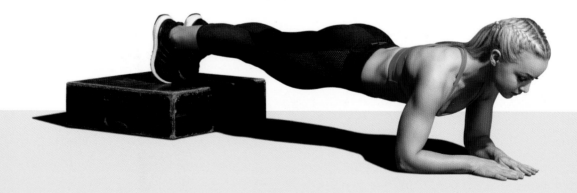

Feet-elevated Side Planks

REPS: 6X30 (3 each side, 30-second – 1-minute rest between each set)

- Place your feet on an elevated platform about a foot off the floor.

- Take your side plank position, so you are in a completely straight line with your head in line.

- Make sure there are no dips in the hips or through the back. Hold the position for 30 seconds.

182

EXERCISE

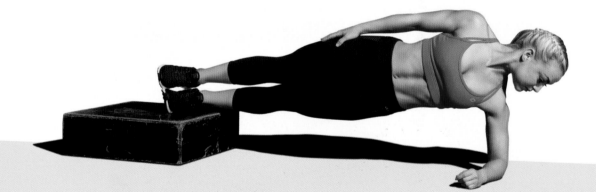

Swiss Ball Knee Tucks

REPS: 3X8-10 (30-second - 1-minute rest between each set)

· Place your knees on your Swiss ball and walk your hands out so that you are in a full plank with your arms extended.

· Bring your knees tightly into your chest and extend back out into your original position.

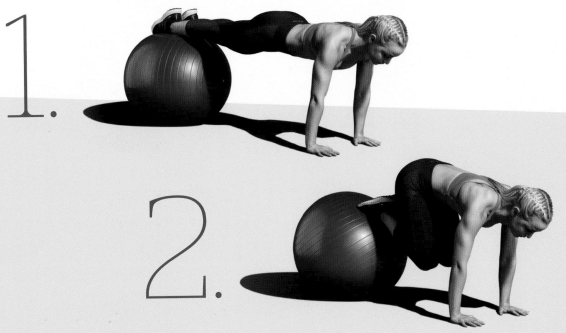

1.

2.

Swiss Ball Pikes

REPS: 3X8 (30-second – 1-minute rest between each set)

· Place your knees on your Swiss Ball and walk your hands out so that you are in a full plank position with your arms fully extended.

· Bend at the hips and draw them upwards so your body pikes, then slowly return to your original plank position.

184

EXERCISE

1.

2.

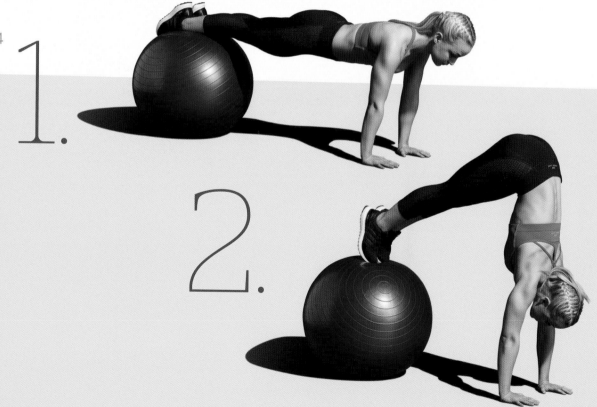

Single-leg Hops

REPS: 3X20 (30-second - 1-minute rest between each set)

- Using your arms, drive up and hop on one leg before taking it back to slightly behind your working leg.

- Repeat 10 times on one leg, then repeat with the other leg leading.

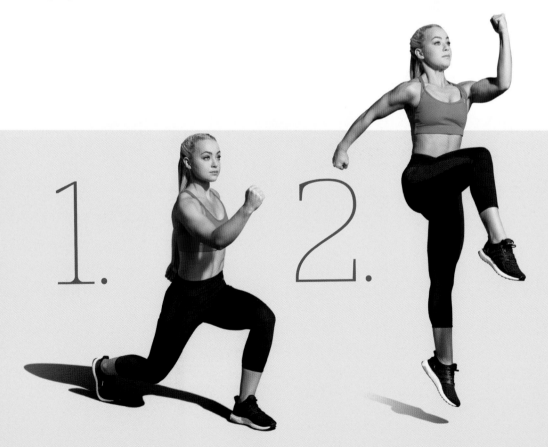

1. 2.

Mountain Climbers

REPS: 3X20 (30-second - 1-minute rest between each set)

· Start in push-up position with arms wider than your shoulders and put your body weight over your hands.

· Take your arms to either side of your chest with your hands facing forwards.

· Bend at the elbow, ensuring your entire body remains completely flat, so no dipping at the hips or through the back. Extend your arms so you make a flat plank.

· Keeping one foot on the floor, bring one knee into your chest, alternating as if running at a quick pace, ensuring your core remains solid and there is no dipping through the pelvis or back.

· Increase your speed, as if you are running on your hands.

186

EXERCISE

1.

2.

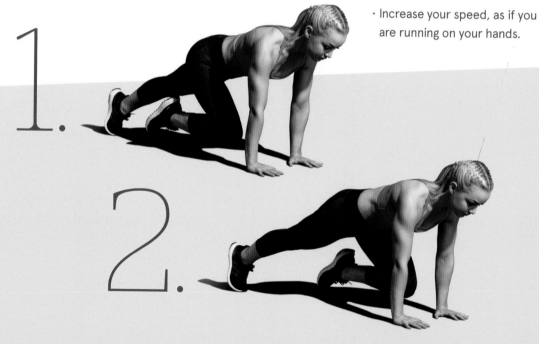

Plank Knee Twists

REPS: 3X20 (30-second rest between each set)

- Assume your plank position with your core tight, your arms extended and your head in line.

- Draw one knee in as close to the opposite side of the body as possible.

- Repeat with the other leg.

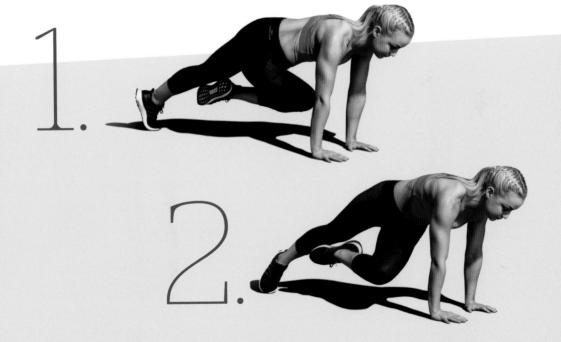

4

The 360
Full-body
Workout

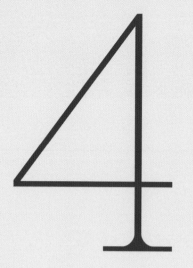

4

The 360 Full-body Workout

The ultimate challenge: an all-over workout designed to get you sweaty and feeling great.

Equipment needed:

 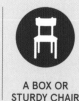

A SWISS BALL | A BOX OR STURDY CHAIR

WARM-UP

Begin with some mobilization and activation of the leg muscles.

Jog on the spot for 3 x 30 seconds/Star Jumps 3 x 20

WORKOUT

Jumping Lunges

REPS: 4X10 (4 each side, 30-second – 1-minute rest between each set)

· As with your Walking Lunges on page 145, remember to keep your chest up and ensure your knees don't roll in or out.

· This time you are going to jump up at the same time as you drop into a lunge.

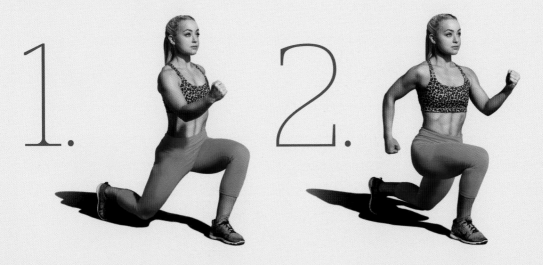

Curtsy Squats with 2-second Pulse

REPS: 4X20 (10 each side, 1-minute rest between each set)

· As if you were going to curtsy, cross one leg behind the other.

· Keep your chest up and pulse for 2 seconds before driving up and repeating on the opposite side.

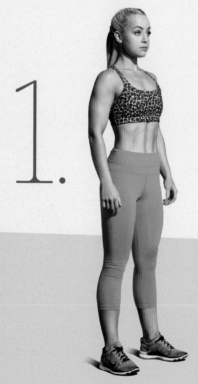

1.

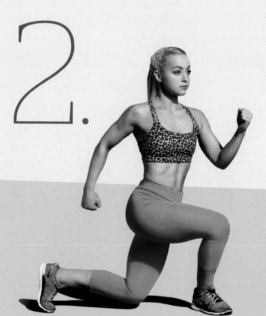

2.

Working hard becomes a habit, a serious kind of fun. You get self-satisfaction from pushing yourself to the limit, knowing that all the effort is going to pay off

Basic Squat

REPS: 4X10 (30-second - 1-minute rest between each set)

· Step your feet slightly wider than hip width apart and have your feet at a comfortable angle, either with toes facing forwards or slightly turned out.

· Keep your chest up. Perhaps aid this by crossing your arms onto your chest.

· Breathe in and lower yourself down (as if you were going to sit on a chair), without your knees rolling in or out and ensuring your heels stay on the ground.

· Bend at both the hips and the knees.

· Once at the bottom of your squat, engage your glutes and legs and drive back up to standing again, avoiding fully locking out the knees or hyperextending (your upper legs should be parallel with the floor and your back should be between a 45- and 90-degree angle to your hips).

194

EXERCISE

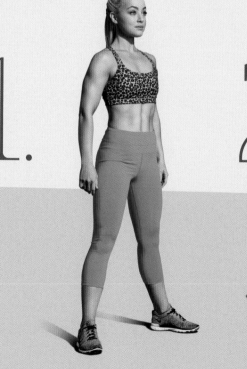

1.

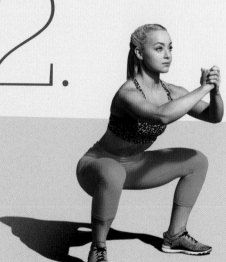

2.

Box Jump onto Platform

REPS: 4X10 (30-second - 1-minute rest between each set)

· Make sure your elevated platform is secure.

· Get into your squat position and drive up to full extension, before jumping onto your sturdy platform.

· Step back down and repeat.

195

EXERCISE

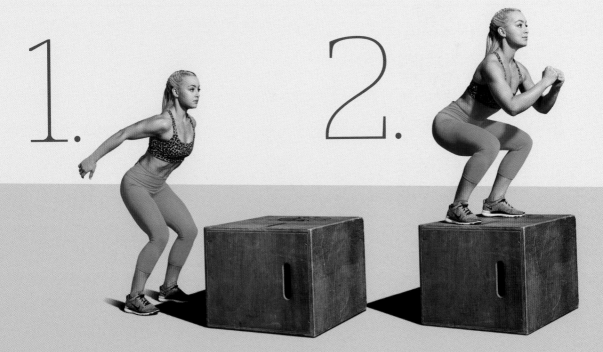

Single-leg Elevated Hip Thrusts

REPS: 4X20 (10 each side, 30-second rest between each set)

· This is the same as the Feet-elevated Glute Bridges on page 146, except this time extend one leg straight ahead so you are now only using one leg, placing the whole foot on the platform.

· Keep your body in line and your core tight so there is no dipping through the hips.

· Drive up using your glutes, before repeating with the other leg.

196

EXERCISE

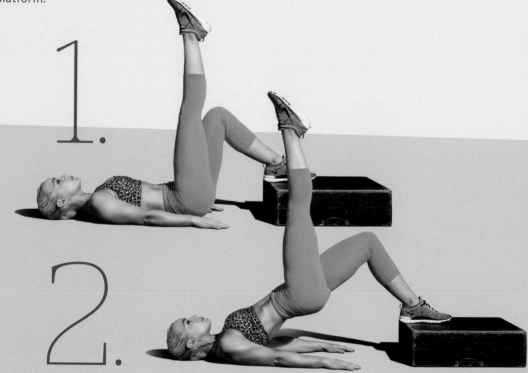

Mountain Climbers

REPS: 4X10 (30-second - 1-minute rest between each set)

· Start in push-up position with arms wider than your shoulders and put your body weight over your hands.

· Take your arms to either side of your chest with your hands facing forwards.

· Bend at the elbow ensuring your entire body remains completely flat, so no dipping at the hips or through the back. Extend your arms so you make a flat plank.

· Keeping one foot on the floor, bring one knee into your chest, alternating as if running at a quick pace, ensuring your core remains solid and there is no dipping through the pelvis or back.

· Increase your speed, as if you are running on your hands.

197

EXERCISE

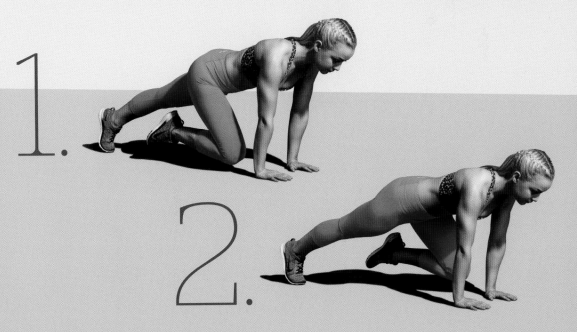

Spider Man Press-ups

REPS: 4X8 (30-second - 1-minute rest between each set)

- After completing the Mountain Climbers on the previous page, drop into the Spider Man Press-up by lowering into a press-up position.

- Bring your left knee to your elbow, then return to your original position when you drive up.

- Repeat on the opposite side.

1.
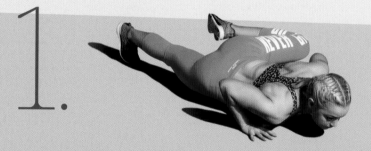

2.
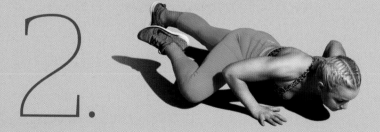

Diamond Press-ups with 2-second Hold (full body or from knees)

REPS: 4X8 (30-second - 1-minute rest between each set)

· Place your hands in a diamond position, so your index finger and thumb are together.

· Keeping your core tight and head in line, lower into your press-up and hold for 2 seconds, before driving up into full extension.

· Repeat as above.

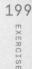

1.

2.

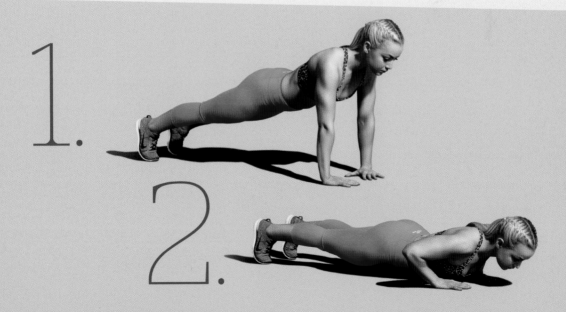

Abdominal Crunches

REPS: 4X10 (30-second - 1-minute rest between each set)

· Lying on your back, bend your knees, with your feet remaining on the floor and place your hands behind your neck to support it.

· Tighten your abs and crunch before returning to your original position.

200

EXERCISE

1.

2.

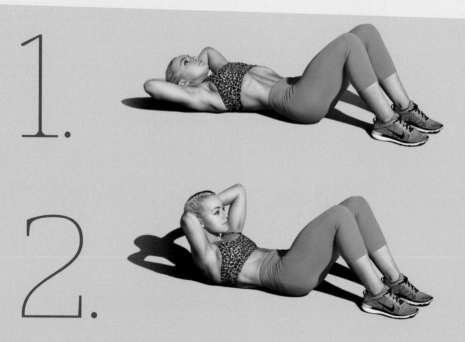

Russian Twists

REPS: 4X12 (6 each side, 30-second - 1-minute rest between each set)

· Sit up with your knees bent and your feet flat on the floor.

· Lean back slightly, keeping your abs tight so you're at an angle.

· Clasp your hands together.

· Twist from side to side, ensuring you keep your head in line and you don't round the lower back.

201

EXERCISE

1.

2.

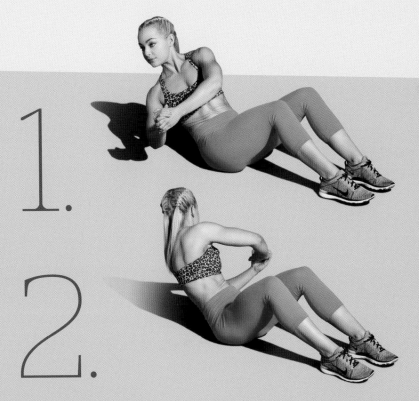

Feet-elevated Plank with Knee Twists

REPS: 3X20 SECONDS (30-second – 1-minute rest between each set)

- Place your feet on an elevated platform, about a foot off the floor

- Assume your plank position with your core tight, your arms extended and your head in line.

- Draw one knee in as close to the opposite side of the body as possible and hold for 20 seconds.

- Repeat with the other leg.

1.

2.

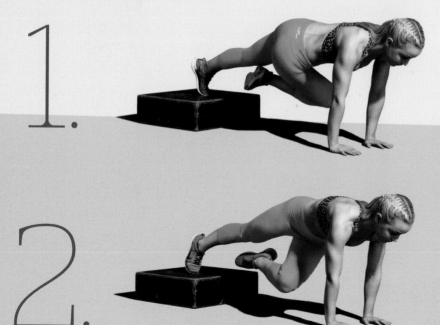

Full-body Burpees

REPS: 3X10 (30-second - 1 minute rest between each set)

· Lying flat face-down on the ground, place your arms stretched above your head.

· Press yourself up into a crouched position and jump upwards before crouching back down.

· Return to your original position with your arms stretched above your head.

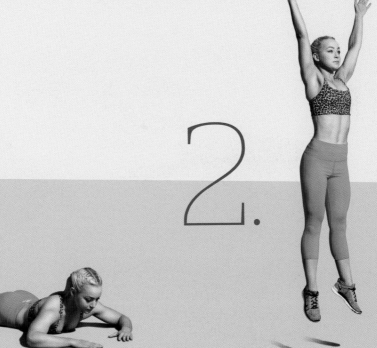

2.

1.

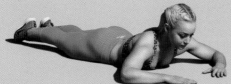

Bunny Hops

REPS: 3X20 (30-second - 1-minute rest between each set)

· Bend down into a crouching position.

· Extend your hands out as far as you can reach.

· Jump your feet in to meet your hands and repeat.

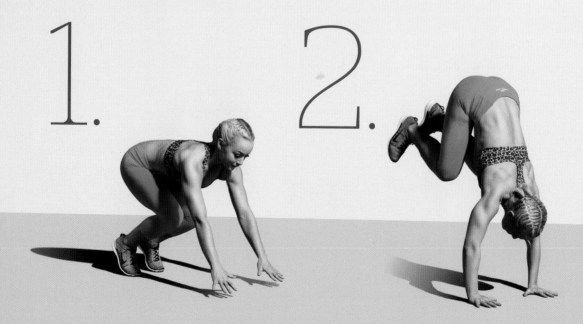

Toe Taps

REPS: 4X20 (30-second - 1-minute rest between each set)

- Using a sturdy chair, stair or box, tap one toe on the chair, then quickly tap the other.

- Use your arms to power you and add speed.

- Keep your chest up.

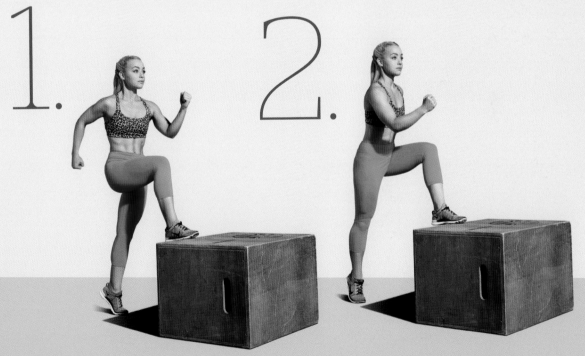

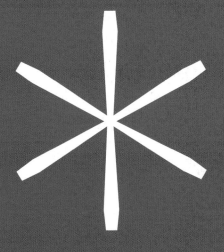

Express Abs

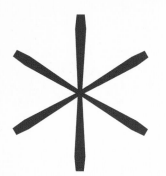

Express Abs

This is perfect for getting in shape pre-holiday, or for keeping your abs fully toned all year round.

Equipment needed:

A SWISS BALL | A BAR BELL | A KETTLE BELL

Swiss Ball Rollouts

REPS: 5X12 (30-second - 1-minute rest between each set)

- Kneeling in front of a Swiss ball, place your forearms and fists on the ball.

- Slowly, and in a controlled manner, roll the ball forwards, straightening your arms and extending your body as far as you can.

- Don't allow your back to sink, or hips to drop.

1.

2.

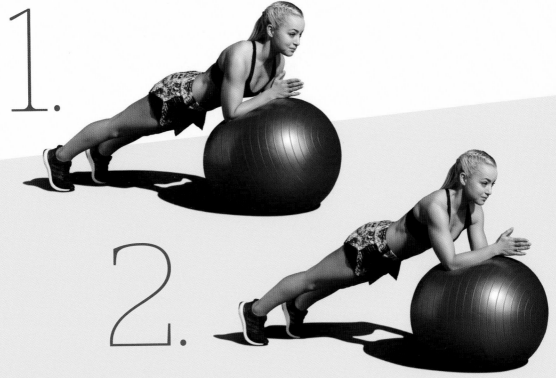

Swiss Ball Pikes

REPS: 5X12 (30-second – 1-minute rest between each set)

- Adopt a press-up position with your hands slightly wider than shoulder width.

- Rest your shins on a Swiss ball, body forming a straight line.

- Without bending your knees, roll the Swiss ball towards your body by raising your hips as high as you can.

- Pause, then return the ball to the starting position by lowering your hips and rolling the ball backwards.

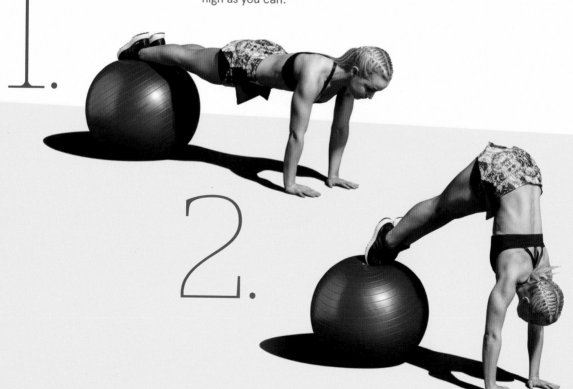

1.

2.

I CAN AND I WILL

Oblique Crunch

REPS: 10X12 (30-second - 1-minute rest between each set)

· Holding a dumbell, sit up with your knees bent and your feet flat on the floor.

· Lean back slightly, keeping your abs tight so you're at an angle.

· Twist from side to side, ensuring you keep your head in line and you don't round the lower back.

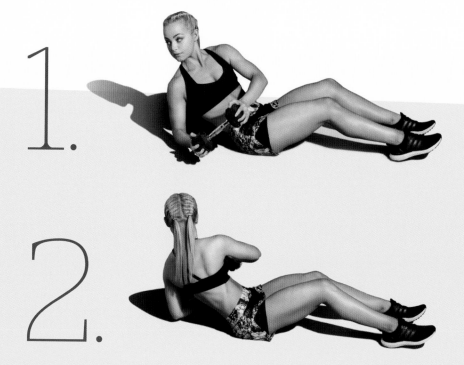

1.

2.

Weighted Crunch

REPS: 10X12 (30-second – 1-minute rest between each set)

- Lying on a mat, feet anchored, make sure your knees are bent with your neck in a neutral position.

- Firmly holding a kettle bell directly above your head, crunch upwards by contracting your abs.

- Hold, then slowly return to the start phase.

1.

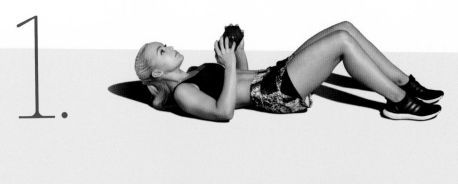

2.

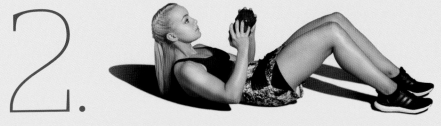

My weekly plan

As we have come to the end of the food and the fitness sections of this book, I thought now would be a good time to share how my typical week looks. I know that starting any kind of regime can feel daunting – any change feels overwhelming – but I did it and so can you.

Obviously I am not at the start of my journey – eating the food in the first half of the book and exercising both in and out of the gym is something I have been doing, consistently, for a long time now. I don't even give it a second thought and I continue to set goals every week that are achievable and that keep me on track. Everything you need to eat well and exercise safely is here. This is your chance to develop lean muscle and see real change in your body.

The aim is change – both mental and physical. The recipes are designed to aid this but the workouts are vital too. Opposite is a typical week for me in terms of exercise – *I am specific, consistent and realistic.*

You shouldn't exercise seven days a week so that you get over-tired or risk injury, but you will need to work out at least four times a week to see results. I have also included two examples of what I do in the gym to give you a proper idea of what a typical week looks like for me. Those of you who follow me on Instagram will know that I have a varied workout routine and enjoy mixing it up when I can.

Monday: Rest day

Incorporating rest days into your week allows your muscles to recover and repair.

Tuesday: Upper body and abs

WARM-UP:
Mountain Climbers (3x20)
Full-body Press-ups (3x8)

WORKOUT:
Neutral-stance Press-ups (3x8)
Shoulder Press-ups (3x8)
Star Twists (4x20)
Tricep Kickbacks (4x10)

FINISHER:
Plank
Lying-down Burpees

Wednesday: Legs

WARM-UP:
Walking Lunges (2x20)
Monster Walks (2x20)

WORKOUT:
Basic Squat with 5-Second Hold (4x12)
Swiss Ball Pikes (3x8)
Single-leg Hops (3x20)
Kettle Bell Deadlift (4x12)

FINISHER:
Jumping Toe Taps (20x4)
Squat Jumps (8-10)

Thursday: Back day (my own programme, not in the book. Gym-based exercise)

Pull-ups (3x6)
Bent-over Row (4x8-10)
Straight-arm Pull-down (4x10)
Lat Pull-down (4x10)
Reverse Flyes (4x10)

Friday: Rest day

Saturday: A full 360 workout

WARM-UP:
Jumping Lunges (4x10)
Star Jumps (3x20)

WORKOUT:
Basic Squat (4x10)
Curtsy Squats with 2-Second Pulse (4x20)
Single-leg Elevated Hip Thrust (4x20)
Box Jump onto Chair

FINISHER:
Full-body Burpees (3x10)
Bunny Hops (3x20)

Sunday: Chest and shoulders (my own programme, not in the book. Gym-based exercise)

Chest Press (4x10)
Arrow Press (4x10)
Cable Flyes (4x10-12)
Lateral Raise (4x12)
Frontal Raise (4x12)
Upright Row (4x10)

Having a healthy mind is just as important as having a healthy body – I truly believe they fuel each other. It's not just about what you feed your body; it's about what you feed your mind and how you care for both.

I talk a lot in this book about how changing my physique helped me achieve a healthy mind - once I'd taken control of a bad situation and decided to make the change, I felt empowered, and I want you to feel the same. Fuelling my body with goodness helped relax my mind and banish the negative thoughts I had to fight against. *The Body Bible* will help you focus on a healthy body image, show you how to cook food you'll enjoy and teach you to love exercise - all of these equate to a happy and positive mindset. I hope I have shown you that it doesn't have to be radical and all at once; it can start with the smallest change, but once you begin you will realize that you are in charge of how you look and feel - and you will understand just how liberating that can be!

Take care of your body – it is the only place you have to live in.

Alice x

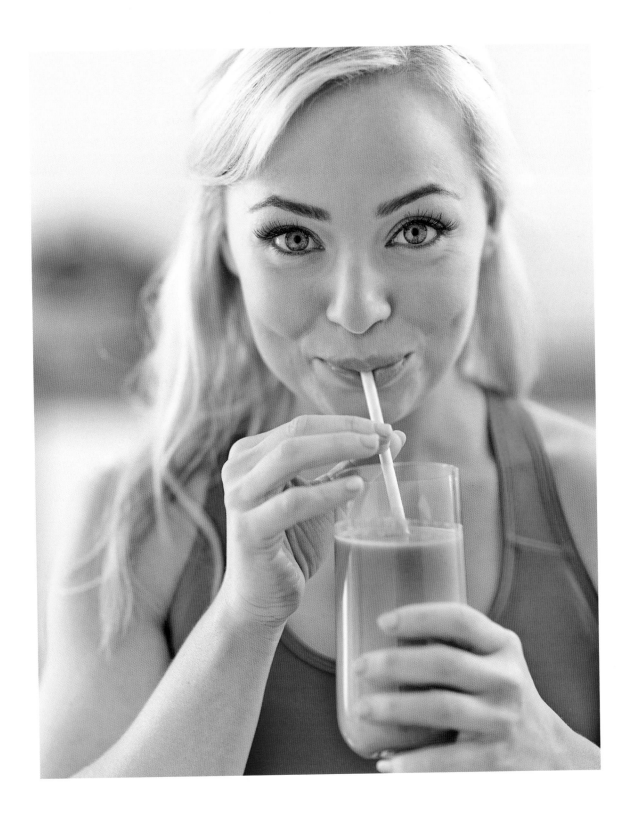

INDEX

ACKNOWLEDGEMENTS

I would firstly like to dedicate this book to everyone who has followed my journey online. You are the people who have made this possible, and you are my daily motivation. I am forever grateful to every single one of you for inspiring me to write this book!

I would also like to thank the boys – James, Tom, Max and Lloyd – from LDN Muscle, without whom I wouldn't be where I am today. They are life-long friends, mentors and people who have inspired me to make a difference within the fitness industry, and for that I am so grateful.

A huge, huge thank you must also go to my wonderful power team: Carly Cook and Becca Barr, two women who have made this dream possible. I would also like to thank my publisher, Carolyn Thorne, and everyone at HarperCollins, who've been there every step of the way to help create this book.

Finally, I want to thank my amazing parents and closest friends, for just always being there, no matter what!